WINNING THE CANCER BATTLE

WINNING THE CANCER BATTLE

nutritional help for breast cancer, prostate cancer, intestinal
cancer, vaginal cancer, and various other cancers

Optimal Health and Wellness Series

Louis Smith
Bob Phillips

ISBN: 1544894473
ISBN 13: 9781544894478
Library of Congress Control Number: 2017904954
CreateSpace Independent Publishing Platform
North Charleston, South Carolina

Winning the Cancer Battle

is presented to you with our sincere desire that it be a rich and valuable source of information, comfort, and encouragement to you, your loved ones, and your friends.

Dedicated to

all determined and passionate individuals who are taking ownership of their lives by dramatically changing their lifestyles and their diets in their efforts to win the cancer battle.

Table of Contents

Part I
Understanding Cancer

Part II
Cancer Prevention

Important Note to the Reader

The information in this book regarding cancer and nutritional supplements is the opinions and ideas of its authors. It should by no means be considered a substitute for the advice of a qualified medical professional. Your doctor should always be consulted before you begin any new diet, exercise, or health-supplement program. Further, the ideas mentioned here are not to be considered diagnosis, prevention, cure, or a prescription to replace a medical doctor's prescribed advice or treatment.

The suggestions of possible supplements that may help various conditions or disorders are for informational purposes only. They are not suggesting dosages, nor are they designed to render a medical diagnosis for readers, their families, or their acquaintances or to render health or professional services. They may be used as a topic of discussion with your medical practitioner.

The authors and the publisher specifically and expressly disclaim any and all liability or responsibility allegedly arising directly or indirectly from the use or application of any information or suggestions contained in this book. Any use of the information in this book is at the reader's discretion.

Pregnant women should not take supplements unless under a doctor's supervision. Again, a health care professional should be consulted regarding your specific situation.

The Death Sentence

Trapped and helpless, I struggled against the ropes that drew me on to death. In my distress I screamed to the Lord for his help. And he heard me from heaven; my cry reached his ears.
—Psalm 18:5–6

"I'm sorry, Louis, but I have some bad news."

My heart was pounding. Deep down I knew what Dr. Naude was going to say.

"We have done everything in our power for your leukemia, and your cancer count keeps rising."

"How much time do you think I have, Doctor?"

"I honestly don't know, Louis. Maybe a number of months. You might be wise to set your affairs in order."

I was twenty-six when that bomb was dropped. LaVerne and I had been married for two years and had a beautiful and bubbly six-month-old daughter. For some time I had not been feeling as vibrant and on top of the world as I used to feel. I was not my usual energetic self, who was always full of life and optimistic about the future.

I did not know I had leukemia at first. All I knew was I started feeling terrible. My weight was dropping. I was listless and had no energy. I realized something was terribly wrong. It bothered me to the point I thought it would be wise to take out a life insurance policy to protect my family.

The insurance company set up the normal physical appointment and did some blood tests. It was at that point the insurance company turned me down. The blood tests revealed I had leukemia. What I'd hoped would be a life policy turned out to be a death sentence.

Thus began my nightmare journey. Over the next few years, I was in and out of hospitals for tests. Medications and blood tests increased. They took so much blood from my arms that they became badly bruised. Eventually they had to take blood from my legs.

As my health began to ebb, so did my attitude. I got mad at God for allowing this to happen to me. I soon started to be grumpy, irritable, and short tempered. My anger spilled over to my family, and I was hard to live with.

Somewhere in this process, I happened to read an article about attitude. It conveyed the idea that you, and you alone, can decide whether you are going to have a good day or a bad day. It went on to say you can wallow in despair or choose to be grateful and rejoice.

A healthy attitude is contagious, but don't wait to catch it from others. Be a carrier.

Well, that day I made a choice. I decided to have a great life as much as possible with the days I had left. I wanted to live my last days to the fullest. I made a decision to fight to live and not to sit down and wait for death to overtake me.

The fight to live turned out to be a war. I tried and experimented with every man-made treatment to stay alive for my wife and child. My doctor aided by pumping in one drug after another in the attempt to find something that might help. The only thing the drugs did was to help destroy my kidneys.

Then a miracle happened.

A friend came into my life and began to tell me about the importance of good nutrition. He talked about whole food supplements and the need for juicing fruits and vegetables. My initial reaction was not positive. I was skeptical. I thought if the importance of good nutrition were true, my doctors, specialists, nurses, and pharmacists would have said something about it. And they hadn't.

That didn't slow down my friend for a minute. He kept talking about the importance of eating food God created rather than just taking drugs. He went on to suggest, "What do you have to lose? You've tried every drug under the sun. Why not try the power of the nutrients in whole foods?" I knew he was right. I'd tried every drug therapy to no avail. I had become a human pincushion for hundreds of needles.

My friend then went beyond just talking about the need for good nutrition. He gave me a two-month supply of juice-extracted, dehydrated, organically grown, nonhybrid, non-GMO, whole food nutrients. LaVerne and I laughed at this. I was already taking pharmaceutical supplements, prescribed and recommended by my doctor. I didn't realize at that time that the pharmaceutical supplements were made from petroleum, turpentine, and synthetic extracts.

Another friend then went so far as to buy me a juicer and a variety of vegetables. He taught me not only how to juice vegetables but also how to make great-tasting smoothies.

In all honesty, I didn't start taking the vitamin supplements or juicing right away. I kept putting it off. However, my friend kept calling to see whether I was feeling any better. He kept reminding me the supplements wouldn't work unless I swallowed them. At some point I must have felt guilty I wasn't taking the supplements, so I started taking them.

A short time after I started taking these supplements, another friend bought me a juicer and a large bag of carrots. He said, "You now don't have any excuse to stay sick." I seemed to be surrounded by people who were willing to share their healthy-living styles with me. I also detoxed: I cut out toxic chemicals (skin creams, shampoos, and laundry detergents and softeners), ate whole food, drank plenty of water, and cut out many sweets and soft drinks.

To my surprise and my doctor's amazement, I began to feel better. My energy level increased. My liver swelling decreased. My internal bleeding stopped. My feet, which looked rotten and smelled terrible, began to heal, and the smell vanished. Also, my terrible body odor disappeared. Within a two-month period, my cancer count was down by nearly 50 percent.

My doctor and I were amazed. How could a simple change of supplement brands do this? When I started taking my friend's supplements, I stopped taking the pharmaceutical-grade vitamins. I also stopped taking the leukemia medications.

After those initial two months and reduction of my cancer count, I began to become very serious about nutrition and health. I started to read about the subject. I went to conferences and listened to tapes and CDs on healthy living. I continued juicing and taking whole food supplements on a regular basis. Thirty-two years have passed since I discovered I had leukemia. Today I'm healthy, vibrant, energetic, positive, and still married, with three healthy grown children and four grandchildren.

I praise God for my near-death situation. Through it I discovered the importance of a nutritionally balanced diet of whole foods, the avoidance of toxins and chemicals, and the need for exercise.

Now, I have dedicated my life to help educate men, women, and young people about the importance of nutrition and healthy living. As you read further in this book, I pray you will be challenged and encouraged to personally experience optimal health for you and your loved ones.

Louis Smith

The longer I live, the more I realize the impact of attitude on life. Attitude, to me, is more important than facts. It is more important than the past, than education, than money, than circumstances, than failures, than successes, than what other people think...or say...or do. It is more important than appearances, giftedness, or skill. It will make or break a company...a church...or a home. The remarkable thing is that we have a choice every day regarding the attitude we will embrace for that day. We cannot change our past. Nor can we change the fact that people will act a certain way. We also cannot change the inevitable. The only thing that we can do is play on the one string we have and that is our attitude. I am convinced that life is 10 percent of what happens to me and 90 percent how I react to it. And so it is with you—we are in charge of our attitudes.

—Chuck Swindoll

Part I
Understanding Cancer

Cancer changes us there's no doubt about that. But it's up to us to decide what that change will mean in our lives, and who we will become as a result.
—Britta Aragon

In 1971, President Richard Nixon declared war on cancer. He alerted the American public to the need of putting forth effort to find a cure for cancer. In 1972, he was successful in having Congress release $1.5 billion for cancer research. By 2009, President Barack Obama directed $10 billion toward health research, with most of it going toward finding a cure for cancer. By 2014, $100 billion worldwide was being given toward cancer research.

Most of the research has been directed toward finding some chemical "magic bullet" that would be able to stop the rising epidemic of cancer. Just think what would happen if some pill or medicine that curbed cancer were discovered. How much would that be worth? The stock in pharmaceutical companies would skyrocket.

Quite often the medical community (traditional medicine) treats the symptoms of diseases rather than the causes of disorders. This treatment focuses on three primary avenues. They are drugs, surgery, and radiation. These treatments are often necessary and beneficial. They are important tools in the doctor's medical bag. Some in the medical community become an expert in one or more of these areas. Traditional medicine has a tendency to view cancer as a hostile invader that comes into the body and that the body has to fight off. Because of this, outside interventions, such as chemotherapy, radiation, and surgery, are necessary.

Many doctors choose to specialize in one area of medicine, such as heart medicine, urinary medicine, or throat medicine. Some doctors enter general practice or family medicine. They may or may not utilize surgery in their practices. The majority of doctors get very little training in drug therapy and almost no education in nutritional health. Most of their drug education comes from the salesmen of the pharmaceutical companies that produce the various drugs. In a recent talk with my doctor, I asked him how much training he received in medical school with regard to nutrition. He said, "I received one class hour."

The only way to keep your health is to eat what you don't want, drink what you don't like, and do what you'd rather not. The average heart specialist can usually check the condition of his patient's heart simply by sending him a bill.
—Mark Twain

When it comes to illness, which do you think is more strategic in the long run: treatment or prevention? When you have a headache, is it because your body has a deficiency in aspirin? When you have colon cancer, is it because you have a deficiency of chemotherapy? When you have breast cancer, is it because you have a deficiency of surgical operations? When you have prostate cancer, is it because you have a deficiency in radiation? Drugs, chemotherapy, surgery, and radiation are only treatments to deal with some disorder. Treatment for various diseases are necessary and important—but what's more important is to attempt to deal with causes of diseases and disorders.

There are more than forty different chemotherapy drugs being used to treat cancer. Chemotherapy consists of heavy metals (poisons) that are designed to kill cancer cells. There are several problems associated with this. The heavy metals kill not only cancer cells but also many healthy cells at the same time. Imagine that. We're going to poison cancer out of the individual.

When the heavy metals of chemotherapy enter the body, the immune system goes into action and attempts to eliminate and remove the heavy metals. Now the body is fighting not only cancer but the chemo drugs also. Sometimes the immune system is so damaged that it is unable to recover from the treatment. This increases the risk of death not just from the cancer but also from other infections that can attack the body. Radiation causes many similar difficulties as chemotherapy.

The side effects of chemotherapy are not pleasant. They include the following:

anemia	dental problems
bleeding	diarrhea
blood count issues	difficulty sleeping
cardiovascular damage	difficulty swallowing
constipation	dry mouth

fatigue	nausea
hair loss	numbness, tingling
mouth sores	taste impairment
infection	vomiting
loss of appetite	weakness

If chemotherapy or radiation is suggested, you would be wise to discuss side effects with your doctor. You might ask whether the drugs or radiation is life threatening or will give you a better quality of life. Of course, you will be interested in discussing your doctor's experience and the survival rates of his or her patients. I doubt whether you'll get a refund from the process if it doesn't work.

You also might ask your doctor about other treatment options. You can ask him or her about his or her views on nutrition and cancer. If your doctor is negative about nutrition or other options, you might ask him or her why. Chemotherapy and radiation are designed to kill cancer cells while nutrition and whole food supplements are designed to boost and strengthen the immune system.

Other follow-up questions might be the following: How much training in nutrition have you received? Would you have your spouse or children go through the same treatment you're recommending for me? How much money will this cost my family? Is it possible for me to get a copy of my medical records when I leave today? You could also broach the subject about getting a second opinion. It's your life your doctor is talking about, you know?

It reminds me of the story of a man who was in the hospital. One day the doctor came into the room and said, "Mr. Jones,

I'm sorry to inform you, but you have only three days to live. Do you have any last requests?"

Mr. Jones responded, "Yes, I would like to see another doctor."

If your doctor is one of the few who become uptight or threatened by these types of questions, you might be wise to seek additional counsel. There are some in the medical profession who view people who ask questions as "poor patients" who will not acknowledge all their great wisdom and expertise. There are others in the medical community who suggest additional factors may be also beneficial, other than drugs, surgery, and radiation. These individuals believe that *alternative medicine* has been shown to produce positive changes in various diseases, including cancer.

Disturbing Discovery
I was stunned to learn that close to 80 percent of the honey sold in the United States is man made.

However, there has been a reluctance by those in *traditional medicine* to accept alternative medicine. They seem to feel that if they do so, they will risk being accused of arousing false hope. Alternative medicine includes acupressure, acupuncture, biofield therapies, chiropractic, heat therapy, homeopathy, lifestyle changes, massage, meditation, mind-body medicine, movement therapy, osteopathy, oxygen therapy, and nutritional therapy with focus on diet changes, herbs, nutrition, vitamins, minerals, and dietary supplements. Alternative cancer therapy is often referred to as *integrative oncology*.

It's our opinion that integrative oncology combines the best of traditional medicine and alternative medicine. It puts together the body's capacity for self-healing with conventional cancer treatments. It's more comprehensive and multidimensional. It's built on a foundation of a healthy diet, positive lifestyle choices, and appropriate supplements.

<u>Traditional Oncology</u>	<u>Integrative Oncology</u>
chemo/surgery/radiation	*nutrition and lifestyle changes*
reactive	preventive
looks at symptoms	looks at underlying causes
prefers isolated treatments	prefers systemic treatments
uses unnatural chemicals	uses natural foods

Numerous studies have been done on cancer and integrative oncology. One study indicated a more than 60 percent reduction in cancer deaths in people who adopted a healthier lifestyle. [1] Another study showed a 68 percent decrease in the risk of dying with the addition of stress-management techniques. [2]

If you have been diagnosed with one of the many forms of cancer, are you choosing to become involved in your health therapy, or have you chosen not to participate? One study suggested that 90 percent of cancers are the result of lifestyle and 5–10 percent are related to inherited genes. [3] Are you satisfied with your lifestyle? Are you fearful? Are you angry? Is there stress in your life? Do you believe you're eating all the daily required nutrition you need? Are you out of shape? Are you getting the exercise you desire? Do you think maybe there might be possible help for cancer treatment other than drugs, surgery, and radiation?

Let's say one day you discover you have mold in the basement of your house. You have several choices. You can choose not to deal with the mold and decide you can live with it the way it is. Or you may determine mold in the basement is not healthy for you or your family. You can decide to scrape the mold off the basement wall and treat it with bleach and other chemicals. When the job of cleaning the wall is finished, you can stand back with pride and look at a clean surface. All is good, right? It is, until a friend informs you that you got rid of the symptoms of the mold but not the cause.

The mold grew because the environment was one of darkness and dampness from moisture on the outside portion of the wall. A small amount of dampness seeped through the wall into the basement to create the perfect condition for mold to grow. The symptoms were dealt with, but not the cause. To deal with the cause, you would need to divert water coming toward the basement wall or cover the wall in some way to prevent moisture from getting into your basement.

Rather than just treating the symptoms of cancer, what do you think are the causes that provided the soil in which your cancer could grow?

Let's take a look at what causes cancer so you can become a participant in your health and move toward the possibility of remission from cancer—or preventing cancer from taking over your body.

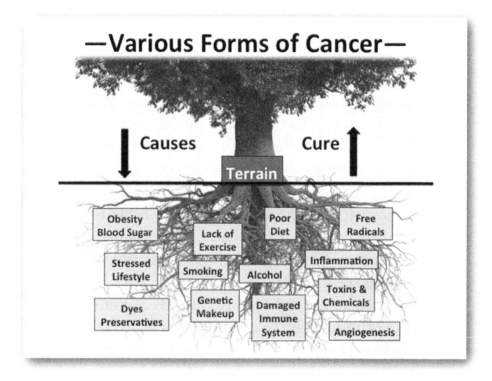

The leaves and branches of the cancer tree represent the various two hundred types of cancer. The *terrain* is the ground from which the cancer grows. The root system indicates the various factors that contribute to the onset of cancer. Any single factor can lead to the presence of cancer, but when they are combined together, the odds of you getting cancer increase dramatically. Remember that 1,688,780 people will hear a cancer diagnosis this year.

- Genetics and family history: 5–10 percent of cancers
- Obesity and dietary habits: 35 percent of cancers
- Environmental influences: 25 percent of cancers
- Lifestyle factors: 30 percent of cancers

To win the battle over cancer, we need to begin to deal with the terrain: the soil, the roots, the environment, and the conditions under which it thrives. If we can change the terrain, we can change the outcome.

In the roots below the tree are thirteen of the most common causes of cancer. The arrow is pointing down toward them. On the right side of the drawing, the arrow is pointing up toward a cure for cancer. To win the battle over cancer, you need to become a participant in the process of healing. You need to begin to fight against the thirteen major causes. It takes courage, determination, and education. Are you ready? Thornton Niven Wilder said, "that every good and excellent thing stands moment by moment on the razor's edge of danger and must be fought for..."

It is courage, courage, courage, that raises the blood of life
to crimson splendor. Live bravely and present
a brave front to adversity!
—Horace

As a participant in your own health, you must understand the concept of cellular health. It's the lack of cellular health that brings about the ravages of cancer and other diseases.

Let's begin with the seven stages of nutrition.

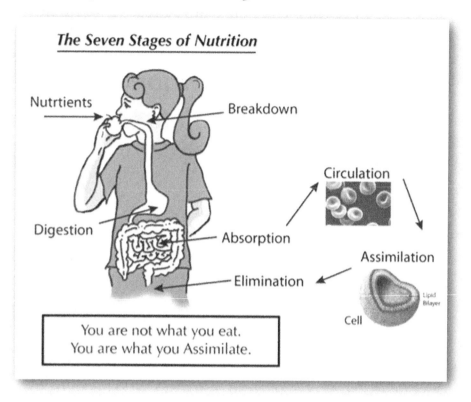

Food and nutrients do not become nutrition until they're broken down in the mouth by chewing and with saliva. A further breakdown of particles takes place in the stomach with various enzymes and acids. The food is then passed to the small intestines to be absorbed into the bloodstream. The food is then taken throughout the entire bloodstream in a process called circulation. This circulation brings all cells in contact with nutrients. As the blood passes by each individual cell, the cell withdraws the nutrients or amino acids needed for its individual cell structure. Different cells have different nutrient needs. Once selected, the nutrients have to then pass through the membrane that covers the cell. It is only when nutrients pass through the cell membrane that you receive nutrition.

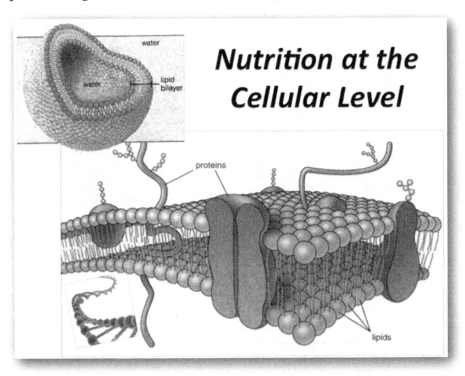

Above is a cutaway of a single cell. The outer membrane is made up of two lipids and a sterol. In the center of the cell is the nucleus, which contains *deoxyribonucleic acid*, or DNA, with genetic information. If the membrane is healthy, it will allow nutrients in to become nutrition. Then the waste products of activity within the cell are ejected through the cell membrane and back into the bloodstream, where they are filtered by the liver and the kidneys and removed from the body through urine flow and solid body waste.

I'm sure you're familiar with the above process—*but here's the catch*. If you don't eat the proper food and nourishment that each individual cell needs, it can become damaged and then easily attacked by the free radicals that are also in the bloodstream. With this thought in mind, you can begin to see the extreme importance of a good diet. If wholesome food does not go into your body, you become the person responsible for your ill health. Later in the book, we will look at nutrients that assist in keeping your cell membrane healthy so it will not be attacked by free radicals.

Disturbing Discovery
I was disappointed to learn that most bacon
and sandwich meats are loaded with nitrates and nitrites,
which can antagonize cancer. I loved these foods, and never
in my battle with cancer had I been warned about this.

Taking care of your health can be likened to taking care of a car. You have a choice when it comes to car care. You can drive your car for quite a long time before it needs oil for lubrication. If you don't add oil when it is needed, the engine will eventually seize up, and you lose the use of the car. You can choose to drive your car in a reckless manner by scratching and denting it. You can drive around with a flat tire. The car still moves, but its efficiency is greatly diminished. The flat tire can lead to further damage if not taken care of.

*The greatest mistake a man can make
is to sacrifice health for any other advantage.*
—Arthur Schopenhauer

Cancer usually doesn't occur immediately. The American Cancer Society informs us that 87 percent of all cancer cases are diagnosed in people fifty years of age or older. For many people it takes from five to twenty years to develop. During that time people drive themselves recklessly through stress, lack of nutrition or poor nutrition, exposure to chemicals and toxins, and lack of proper exercise and rest. Eventually their bodies begin to break down and lose efficiency. Then they go to the doctor (the body mechanic) for a magic pill to instantly change what has taken years to cause.

In the chapters ahead, we will be looking at the importance of the immune system. We will examine the causes of cancer. We will consider the benefits of supplements and the effects of synergy. We will suggest healthy diet changes. We will stress the importance of exercise. And we will discuss the effects of cancer as they relate to the mental, emotional, and spiritual life of the cancer patient and his or her family.

We will also share a number of stories about people who encountered cancer and how they dealt with it. Their experiences are not a formal medical presentation but something they personally encountered. Their testimonies are included to create an attitude of hope and inspiration in the reader.

No one can predict precisely the path that cancer will lead him or her down. Some have found remission and healing. Others and their families had to face the last human encounter with courage and acceptance.

We cannot give you absolute guarantees that you will escape the ravages of cancer. Only God can do that. We will, however, suggest a plan for healthy living that will make it more difficult for cancer to have free rein in your body. To win the battle over cancer, you must understand cellular health. Since cells become damaged by free radicals, the question arises, is there any way to protect our cells? The answer lies in understanding our immune system and how the food in our diets helps our bodies to protect our cells. Join us in this adventure.

When I was forty-nine, the doctors discovered I had liver cancer. They sent me home with no treatment and told me my cancer was too advanced to give me chemotherapy. Realizing my life had been taken away from me, I became sad, frustrated, and desperate.

That's when I talked with Louis. He suggested we try the same thing he did for his leukemia. He suggested a detox program, juicing with fresh vegetables (especially carrots) daily. I also began to eliminate *systemically* applied pesticides (through the roots) from my diet. I started using organic vegetables and washing off sprayed-on pesticides. I used a vegetable-cleaning product called Green to break down the surfactants that hold pesticides onto the leaves of vegetables.

I basically began a raw-food diet. I also cut out sugars, meat, and acid foods. I started a daily regimen of whole food supplements and discontinued the nutrients made from petroleum and turpentine.

I stopped purchasing store-bought juices and began to eliminate fried foods and margarines. All these changes were not easy and took a little while to accomplish, but I was determined to try to extend my life beyond the dismal prognosis of my doctors.

I began drinking protein shakes, and to my amazement I started feeling better by the day. My energy level increased, and the yellowing in my skin vanished. It wasn't long before I was up and out of bed. When I went to my doctor for the next visit, he was absolutely amazed at how well I had become. That was twenty-five years ago.

Unfortunately, after being cancer-free for over twenty years, my cancer returned. I knew it was my fault. I had gotten back into all my old habits of enjoying chocolates, drinking store-bought fruit juices and coffee, and enjoying sweets and fried and smoked foods.

This time the cancer came on with a vengeance. It started in my womb and then spread to other internal organs. The doctors tried every man-made cure. They operated and then informed me I was too weak for chemotherapy.

At seventy-five years of age, I felt terrible. I was tired and desperately ill. I was too weak to get out of bed. That's when my son arrived from the United States with a juicer. He helped me get on track. I started juicing again with lemons and carrots and other organic fruits and vegetables. He also put me on massive amounts of whole food supplements and antioxidants. Within days I was feeling better. My energy level increased, and the next time I went to the doctor, he said I was on my way to recovery.

It's now been over five years since I conquered stage 4 cancer for the second time. I'm so impressed with God's way of healing the body with whole food supplements and juicing of vegetables.

The human body essentially recreates itself every six months.
Nearly every cell of hair and skin and bone dies
and another is directed to its former place.
You are not who you were last November.
—Donald Miller

Our immune system has been designed by God to recognize healthy cells and tissues and, at the same time, attack invaders. These invaders take the form of foreign substances, like viruses, bacteria, protozoa, fungi, yeast, free radicals, pesticides, environmental toxins, heavy metals, dyes, food colorings, and chemicals. The organs of the immune system include bone marrow, the thymus gland, the spleen, and the lymph nodes.

The thymus gland is a small organ that rests above the heart and behind the sternum, in the chest. This gland somehow teaches white blood cells how to identify and destroy foreign invaders in the body.

The spleen is about the size of your fist. It's located in the upper-left quadrant of the abdomen, behind the stomach. It functions as a filter for the bloodstream as it destroys old or dead blood cells and helps remove them from the body.

The lymph system has many channels throughout the body. It has from five hundred to seven hundred lymph nodes, where toxins and other waste materials from cells gather and are eliminated. The greatest collections of lymph nodes are found in the groin, neck, and underarms. This unique system does not have any pumping organ like the heart. It relies on the smooth movement of fluids assisted by the pressure created by muscle movement and the beating of the heart.

The lymph system can be likened to a sewer system for a busy city. It drains all the waste materials produced by every cell within the body. You should be very grateful for this God-designed system. If it did not operate properly, we would die in our own waste. If you never flushed your toilet at home, sewage would spill over onto the floor and create a tremendous mess. It would take much work to clean up such a tragedy. The spleen and lymph nodes act as the filtering garbage dumps for the waste products from the war on invaders.

Disturbing Discovery
*I was stunned to discover rats could live longer
if they ate the cardboard cereal container of some brands
than if they ate the actual cereal in the box.*

Often, the immune system is compared to a protective army. Your body's first line of defense starts with your skin, which keeps many foreign substances from entering. It's followed by hairs in the nose, which act as small barriers to stops some bacteria. Then there is the wall of mucous membranes that wash out microbes by the use of nasal drippings, saliva, coughing, sneezing, tears, and vaginal secretions. The linings of your intestines also help create a barrier from the outside world into the body.

Your body also houses billions of foreign soldiers called "friendly" or "good" bacteria. They are housed in your intestines. These friendly bacteria aid in digestion, produce vitamins and energy for the body, stimulate bowel contraction, and help defend the body by gobbling up the soldiers of "unfriendly" or "bad" bacteria that invade your body.

As was mentioned earlier, the human body is made up of fifty to a hundred trillion cells. What is a mindblower is that you have more bacteria in your body than you have body cells. It's estimated that the normal gut of an adult houses about four pounds of good and bad bacteria. Good and bad bacteria are constantly coming into our bodies and going out of our bodies. When you sit on the toilet and eliminate solid waste, it's estimated that each pound of waste leaving your colon contains unabsorbed food matter and about fifty billion bacteria.

Many people take probiotics (*acidophilus*) to replenish good bacteria in their intestinal systems. One study indicated that probiotics improved the immune system along with assisting the increase of natural killer cells. [1]

Antibiotics were created to assist the body in fighting infections the immune system is having difficulty in dealing with. Their main function is to kill bad bacteria. They are often quite successful in helping the body rid itself of disease-causing bacteria. Antibiotics are useless against viruses.

In the process of killing bad bacteria, antibiotics also kill beneficial bacteria. The loss of beneficial bacteria can lead to fungal infections. I have a friend that was dealing with a urinary infection. The doctors were giving him many doses of antibiotics, to no avail. For more than a year, he was dealing with pain and discomfort.

I shared with him that often people who have urinary infections also have a loss of healthy bacteria in their intestines. I suggested that he would be wise to cut back on his intake of sugar and white breads. As a result of our talk, he decided to take some probiotics to add back healthy bacteria. He also began taking garlic with allium. Two weeks later he called me and said that this was the best he had felt in a year and a half. He was now off antibiotics and was attempting to cut back on sweets, which, he said, was very difficult. So what else is new?

Also housed in your intestines are billions of your immune cells. Their job, along with that of the friendly bacteria, is to seek out and destroy foreign matter from penetrating the intestinal wall of defense. It's estimated that more than 70 percent of immune cells are housed in the digestive tract. When foreign substances break through the outer defense wall of your nose, lungs, or intestines, the battle for your health increases dramatically.

Your body's immune soldier cells have a very sophisticated communication system with one another. They are also organized into different divisions and have assigned duties. Your white blood cells are referred to as immune cells. Their birthplace is your bone marrow. The duty of these white cells, or T cells, is to patrol the bloodstream. They are the interior front line of defense in preventing germs from gaining a foothold. Once birthed, they move to the thymus gland, where they mature before entering the bloodstream. While in the thymus gland, they are educated, so to speak, as to their specific roles. There are millions of these soldiers in each drop of blood.

These T cells put out a communication warning when something is wrong in your body. They are a seek-and-destroy unit. They have the ability track down enemy pathogens. They also have the ability to shoot *gamma interferon* into a terrorist invader like a poisonous dart.

Helper T cells are the emergency alarm system. They produce *interleukin*, which helps produce an inflammatory response to damaged tissue or cells under attack. They instruct B cells to produce antibodies in response to invading viruses, bacteria, fungi, yeast, and parasites.

Another division is called B cells. They specialize in identifying and marking particular enemy invaders in your blood and lymph so cells known as *phagocytes* can easily identify them. B cells produce antibodies matched to specific antigens. These cells have a memory of the enemy invaders they have encountered in the past and their chemical makeups. They can call up the necessary antigen needed to defeat them if they attack again. They have the ability to poke holes in germs, which causes them to sort of bleed to death. Phagocytes love to engulf and digest the antigens.

Natural killer cells are an elite type of immune cell. They can recognize cancerous and infected cells and destroy them instantly. They are armed with an estimated hundred different biochemical poisons that can destroy the enemy invaders.

There are other immune cells, such as *cytotoxic T cells, suppressor T cells, phagocytes, granulocytes,* and *macrophages.* They also assist in digesting many viruses, bacteria, and old and dead cells.

It has been said that an army travels on its stomach. Soldiers in any battle need proper food and nourishment to put forth the energy necessary to fight and endure. The same is true for the immune system. Later in the book, we will examine nutrients that can boost the immune system by 37 percent in as little as twenty days.

Cancer is a multidimensional battle
against a mammoth opponent.

A Balanced Immune System = Optimal Effectiveness

Internal Threats	External Threats	Cancer	Infection
Arthritis	Allergies	Hepatitis	Bacteria
Lupus	Eczema	HIV	Mold
Diabetes	Asthma	Shingles	Fungus
Crohn's	Sinusitis	TB	Viruses

Immune Over-reaction   Immune Under-reaction

Optimal Effectiveness

Having struggled with headaches for most of my life, I thought they were something I would just have to put up with. In spite of the headaches, I graduated near the top of my class in high school and then went across country to New York City for college.

Once I graduated with my BA, I came back home to Southern California. It was at this time my headaches began to get progressively worse. I went to the doctor a half a dozen times but with no answer to my pain. Finally, in February 2011, I was able to see a wonderful doctor. He would become the man who saved my life. After a brief appointment with him, he concluded that a CT scan of my head was necessary.

Within an hour of my scan, he made a phone call that would change my life forever. He was calling to let me know he had found the problem. He had discovered a mass on my brain. The tumor had likely been growing my whole life. It was life-threateningly huge—7.8 centimeters, to be exact. I was just twenty-five years old when I went into my first of many brain surgeries. I remained in the hospital for thirty-three days after that first surgery.

The mass was benign, however, and I didn't require chemotherapy or radiation. The removal of the mass left a large gaping hole. I began to have a plethora of problems, with the struggle of my memory being the worst.

Before I got sick, I was planning to go to law school. After my diagnosis I was unsure whether I would ever live independently again. That was until I was introduced to taking whole food supplements.

A childhood friend who had lost his father to a brain tumor several years prior contacted me. He had been involved in taking whole food supplements and was reaping the life-changing benefits from cellular nutrition.

I began taking small amounts of vitamins, minerals, and protein shakes. Within just a few months, I started noticing changes. I was feeling more alert and "clear." My memory was slowly beginning to get better, although it was a work in progress. I didn't feel nearly as foggy as I had felt after the tumor.

I was amazed at the benefits I felt with whole food supplements, especially considering the small amount of product I was taking in such a small span of time. It was truly a miracle. I believe with all my heart that whole food nutrition and eating foods in the way they were created were central to my health.

Today, I'm doing well. I'm working and hopefully attending graduate school this year. I still have a few struggles, but God is good. He's always good and always faithful. I firmly believe that food was created to nourish, sustain, and heal our bodies.

Feed your faith and your fears will starve to death…and
remember scars are tattoos with better stories.

N o one ever looks forward to hearing the words "You've got cancer." It's the most dreaded disease in America. The American Cancer Society informs us that in 2017, an estimated 1,688,780 new cases of cancer will be diagnosed. They also state an estimated 606,920 people will die from various forms of cancer. It's even possible that you could be one of them.

Many people who are informed they have cancer believe they are now at the mercy of their surgeons, radiation oncologists, medical oncologists, and chemotherapy nurses. They're not aware of other ways to approach their cancer.

Have you ever wondered exactly what cancer is and where it comes from? Let's start by examining what cancer is not. It's not contagious. There are no cancer "carriers." No one can give you cancer. There are no cancer parasites or cancer viruses. Also, there are no cancer bacteria or cancer fungi. However, parasites, viruses, bacteria, and fungi can play a negative role in causing the body to struggle with cell damage.

Most people who encounter cancer believe they're *victims* of the dreaded disease. It's sort of as if cancer has just suddenly come upon them from out of the blue. The unfortunate truth is they're not victims but participants in the disease. Remember that only 5–10 percent of cancers are genetically triggered; the majority, 90–95 percent, are caused by diet and lifestyle. Diet and lifestyle are things we can begin to control. The shocking truth is that we participate in the onset of cancer. This book is written with the intent to help motivate you to become involved in prevention of the dreaded disease.

Disturbing Discovery
I was horrified to discover that a university study in 2013 found that up to 69 percent of the imported olive oil labeling in the popular brands they tested was false.

Cancer starts in cells that have been attacked or damaged by *free radicals*. Everyone is exposed to these molecules on a daily basis. Free radicals are atoms or molecules that are missing an electron. Usually, electrons travel in pairs. The free radical does not have paired electrons. When it comes into contact with another molecule, it attempts to steal or pull away an electron from the normal or healthy molecule, thus making it unstable or damaged. When this damage or stealing happens in healthy cells, they then reproduce or mutate other unhealthy cells—and a chain reaction continues. As the number of unhealthy cells grows, they begin to form small tumors. A tumor is an abnormal growth or swollen mass of tissue. This mass of tissue is made of damaged cells.

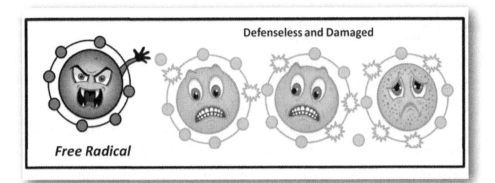

For a microtumor to become dangerous, it needs to create a new network of blood vessels to feed it. This is made possible as the damaged cells produce chemical substances called *angiogenins.* An angiogenin is a small single-chain protein that stimulates the formation of new blood vessels.

Benign tumors are local and grow but do not spread to other areas. Malignant tumors are masses of cancerous cells. They are invasive and out of control. They can spread throughout the body, especially if they get into the lymphatic system. This spreading is called *metastasis.* It's a complex process involving the spreading of a cancer to distant parts of the body from its original site. New studies indicate that 60–70 percent of patients have initiated the metastatic process by the time of their cancer diagnosis. [1]

Hyperplasia takes place when normal cells mutate or divide at a rapid pace and cause a crowding effect. An example of this takes place in the prostate organ of men. It's called *benign prostatic hyperplasia or hypertrophy*, or BPH for short.

It's estimated that the human body contains from fifty to a hundred trillion cells, depending on the size of the person.

Cells replace themselves at different rates, from a few hours to a few months. Skin and nerve cells live for longer periods.

When it comes to BPH in a man's prostate, the cells are reproducing more rapidly than they're dying off. This causes a crowded condition. The urethra passes through the prostate and gets squeezed because of this crowding. This squeezing creates a smaller urine flow and lengthened time in emptying the bladder. BPH is not considered cancer, but it can lead to cancer.

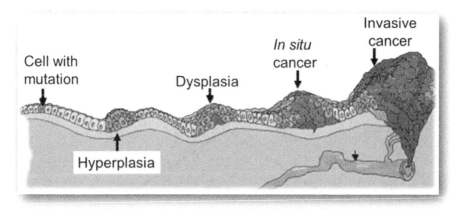

Free radicals come from three major areas:

External factors include water pollution, air pollution, chemicals, pesticides and herbicides, UV light, and radiation.

Internal factors include genetics, infections, inflammation, and DNA damage by free radicals, dyes, and preservatives.

Lifestyle factors consist of things like unhealthy diet, obesity, sun exposure, stressed lifestyle, lack of exercise, alcohol, and smoking and chewing tobacco. It is estimated that there are over four thousand different chemicals in cigarette smoke, and over forty of them are cancer producing. It's also estimated that our cells encounter ten thousand free radical attacks a day.

Antioxidant armies within our bodies deal with most of these free radical attacks.

There are two primary ways doctors and the public describe cancer. Either they refer to the organ that has cancer in it, or they describe it by the cell or tissue that's involved.

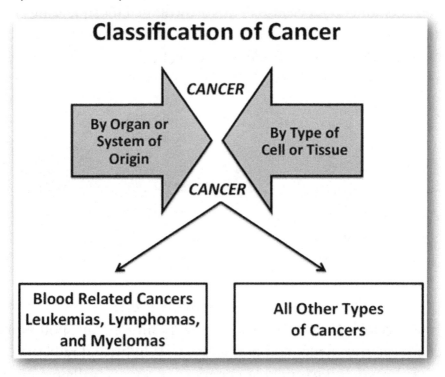

Carcinomas are cancers that affect the skin, mucous membranes, glands, and internal organs. Carcinomas are the most common cell type of cancer, accounting for 80–90 percent of cancers. These cancers arise in cells called *epithelial cells*. Epithelial cells include the cells of the skin and those that line body cavities and cover organs.

Sarcomas are cancers that affect muscles, connective tissue, and bones.

Lymphomas are cancers that affect the lymphatic system.

Myelomas are cancers of the cells in the immune system.

Leukemias are cancers of blood-forming tissue, often referred to as blood cancer.

Mixed types are cancers of cells with different characteristics.

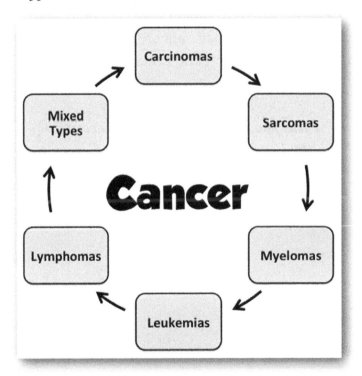

The American Cancer Society suggests that 50 percent of men and 33 percent of women will encounter some form of cancer during their lifetimes. There are over two hundred different types of cancers.

The Most Common Cancers

bladder cancer

blood cancer

bone cancer

brain cancer

breast cancer

cervical cancer

colon cancer

endocrine cancer

esophageal cancer

gastric cancer

head and neck
cancer

kidney cancer

liver cancer

ovarian cancer

pancreatic cancer

prostate cancer

respiratory cancer

skin cancer

testicular cancer

thyroid cancer

uterine cancer

Disturbing Discovery
I was shocked to discover that according
to the Environmental Working Group, the
most pesticide-ridden food is strawberries.

Cancer signs refer to factors on the body that can be visually seen by doctors and others. They include things like lumps, moles, rashes, dark spots, coughing, fast breathing, and fever.

Cancer symptoms, on the other hand, are sometimes experienced or seen only by the individual. They might involve blood in the stools or urine, dizziness, stomach disorders, throat discomfort, decreased urine flow, and aches and pains.

Listed below are signs and symptoms that could indicate the possibility of cancer. You would be wise to consult your doctor, and he or she will help you determine whether the sign or symptom indicates cancer or some other disorder you may be experiencing.

1. Changes in bowel or bladder habits and blood in stools or urine could indicate bladder, urinary, or rectal cancers.
2. Depression sometimes indicates the possibility of pancreatic cancer.
3. Difficulty swallowing is often related to throat cancer.
4. Fatigue, or extreme tiredness, can be related to a number of different cancers.
5. Fever might indicate the presence of blood-related cancers like leukemia.

6. Hoarseness can signal lung cancer or thyroid cancer.
7. A lump or area of thickening that can be felt under the skin relates to breast cancer or testicular cancer.
8. Persistent cough or trouble breathing is often indicative of respiratory cancer.
9. Persistent indigestion or discomfort after eating points to the possibility of stomach or intestinal cancer.
10. Persistent lower-back pain sometimes indicates the presence of kidney cancer.
11. Persistent, unexplained fevers or night sweats could be related to blood cancers.
12. Persistent, unexplained muscle or joint pain can represent some type of bone or muscle cancer.
13. Skin changes, such as yellowing, darkening, or redness of the skin, sores that won't heal, or changes to existing moles point to skin or oral cancers.
14. Unexplained bleeding or bruising of the skin can indicate skin cancer.
15. Unexplained weight changes, including unintended loss or gain, can be related to pancreatic, stomach, or esophagus cancers.
16. Unusual bleeding or discharge often accompanies colon, rectal, or breast cancers.

Keep in mind that just because you might have one or more of these signs, it does not mean you have cancer. They are simply signs that accompany cancer. It's important that you let your doctor know the signs and symptoms you're experiencing. In that way he or she can make a more informed diagnosis of what might be ailing you.

Cancer is, in reality, a life-and-death issue for many people. It immediately strikes fear because the average cancer patient has only a 60 percent chance of surviving the next five years. (2) It's estimated that this disease will take one in four people. To put it in perspective, over sixteen hundred people a day die of some form of cancer. It's second only to heart disease.

Cancer is a formidable and challenging illness. It's costly not only physically but also financially, mentally, and emotionally. It's no wonder that many people experience anger, anxiety, fear, and even panic when they hear the big *C* word. But they're not alone. Their families and friends also experience many of the same emotions. It's hard not only on the individuals with cancer. Their caregivers go through the same fears and often have to pick up the financial pieces after their loved ones die, along with dealing with the emotions of loss. When children get cancer, their parents also suffer with them. Parents don't want to outlive their own children. According to the American Cancer Society, "After accidents, cancer is the second leading cause of death in children ages 1 to 14." (3) Each year there seems to be an increase of childhood cancers.

Kern Reddel's Story as told by Anne Reddel

In October, Ken was diagnosed with non-Hodgkin's lymphoma in the chest. After six months of chemotherapy and radiation, along with all the unpleasant and unwanted side effects, his disease went into remission. Ken was told, after five years of follow-up, that he was cured.

Imagine our surprise when eleven years later, in June, he had a growth at the back of his throat removed and we were told that it was non-Hodgkin's lymphoma again! Fortunately, this time it was low grade—but unfortunately, three other tumors were also found, several quite large.

After several months of monitoring, it was decided by the doctors that chemotherapy should be commenced as the tumors were increasing in size. We thought, "Oh no, not chemotherapy again!"

In the meantime, Ken had been introduced to a product that contained carotenoids, flavonoids, and cruciferous nutrients. Ken started using these totally natural products in September on a double dose. Ken decided to increase the dose to four packs daily.

Amazing things began to happen!

The smallest tumor totally disappeared in four to five weeks. The middle egg-shaped tumor disappeared in about two and a half months. The largest tumor (which could be monitored only by CT scan) was proven to be totally resolved last week! This was with no chemotherapy!

Ken took those fantastic phytonutrients along with a variety of other vitamins and minerals. He also took a protein shake, and his immune system has responded by getting rid of the tumors.

Part II
Cancer Prevention

We may never understand illnesses such as cancer.
In fact, we may never cure it. But an ounce of prevention
is worth more than a million pounds of cure.
—David Agus

As a general rule, most physicians deal with symptoms of cancer rather than the causes. They are trained to look for the typical signs of any disorder or disease. Often it's the patient who complains of lumps, moles, and dark spots on his or her body. Or the patient might mention a stomach disorder or a throat discomfort or that he or she feels tired all the time. The doctor then proceeds to identify symptoms, which often represent a particular disorder. This process is quite normal and understandable. Hippocrates, the father of medicine, suggested that it is good to listen to the person who is hurting for he or she will tell you what is wrong with him or her.

The doctor will then suggest a prescription of rest, drugs, and/or medical tests—and a follow-up visit. The doctor might suggest chemotherapy, surgery, or radiation. It's doubtful you will hear most doctors say, "You're overweight and you need to go on a diet" or "You're eating too much sugar" or "You need to start reading labels of the food you're putting in your body" or "Your lifestyle is very stress producing. You need to sit down, get organized, and get your act together" or "You worry too much" or "You're an angry person. What's going on in your life?" or "You're falling apart. You need some exercise" or "How's your mental, emotional, and spiritual life doing at this time?" That would be a shock if he or she started mentioning things like, "It's not what you're eating that's the problem; it's what's eating you."

In the pages following, we will attempt to address the terrain or environment where the seeds of cancer begin. Remember that healthy cells resist cancer and other diseases.

Disturbing Discovery
I was shocked to discover that certain foods
are enriched with turpentine, rocks, and metal filings.

The Center for Disease Control informs us that 480,000 people a year die from smoking—and 41,000 of those die from breathing secondhand smoke. Smoking harms nearly every organ in your body.

Smoking is tied to bladder cancer, esophageal cancer, laryngeal cancer, lip cancer, mouth cancer, throat cancer, tongue cancer, and lung cancer. Ninety percent of lung-cancer deaths are due to smoking.

There is a smoking link with other disorders and complications:

appetite suppressant	COPD	risk of heart disease
asthma	coughing	stained teeth
bad breath	habit formation	tuberculosis
bronchitis	pneumonia	yellow fingers
cataracts	pregnancy difficulties	

Smoking is one of the leading causes of preventable death. The mortality rate among smokers is three times higher than it is among nonsmokers. It's been said that smoking won't send you to hell; it just makes you smell as if you've been there. If you want to shorten your life-span and the life-spans of those around you, and if you would like some of the complications mentioned above, just ignore our comments.

Over 36 percent of American adults are losing the battle with obesity. There are 12.7 million children and adolescents that are considered obese. The medical costs for obesity are a staggering $147 billion a year. (1)

For men with excess weight, their chances of dying of prostate cancer are increased by 34 percent. For overweight women, their chances of dying from breast cancer double. As little as five to ten pounds of excess weight increases the risk by 20 percent, and forty to fifty pounds of excess weight doubles the risk of breast cancer. (2)

One of the reasons for excessive weight gain can be attributed to the serving of larger portions. Twenty years ago you would be served a three-inch bagel with 140 calories. Today, bagels are six inches and contain 350 calories—an increase of 210 calories. When you ordered french fries twenty years ago, they were served in a 2.4-ounce bag with 210 calories. Today, the bag holds 6.9 ounces with 610 calories—an increase of 400 calories. A box of Chinese rice and vegetables twenty years ago held two cups and contained 435 calories. Today, the same meal is served in a box and holds 4.5 cups with 865 calories—an increase of 430 calories.

Children are always being told to eat more by parents who are always being told to eat less.

Another factor in obesity is the poor choice of foods that are eaten. Snack foods like Twinkies, Ding Dongs, Hostess CupCakes, and various cookies, chips, and so on are on the rise. According to a Nielsen Report, snack foods are a $374 billion industry.

Patrick Quillin, in his book *Beating Cancer with Nutrition*, lists the "average annual consumption of low-nutrient foods:

756 doughnuts
60 pound cakes & cookies
23 gallons of ice cream
7 pounds of potato chips
22 pounds of candy
200 sticks of gum
365 cans of soft drinks
90 pounds of fat
140 pounds of sugar" [3]

The Ex-Dieter's Psalm

My stomach is my shepherd;
I shall not want low-calorie foods.
It maketh me to munch on potato chips and bean dip;
It leadeth me into 31 Flavors;
It restoreth my soul food.
It leadeth me in the paths of cream puffs in bakeries.
Yea, though I waddle through the valley of the shadow of
dieting,
I will fear no skimmed milk;
For my appetite is with me;
My Twinkies and Ding Dongs, they comfort me;
They anointeth my body with calories;
My scale tippeth over!
Surely chubbiness and contentment shall follow me
All the days of my life.
And I shall dwell in the house of Marie Callender's Pies
forever.
Never eat more than you can lift.
—Miss Piggy

Obesity has a strong relationship with the following:

cancer	depression	erectile dysfunctions
fatty liver disease	high blood pressure	sleep apnea
gallstones	high cholesterol	stroke
guilt	joint problems	trouble breathing
heart disease	low self-image	type 2 diabetes

An inactive lifestyle with a lack of exercise is another strong factor in obesity. This is true for not only adults but also children. Many children who used to go outside to play now stay inside and watch television and play video games.

It may be the right time for you to take some serious time to think about any extra weight you've been carrying. Are you happy with your present weight? When you look in the mirror, do you say, "Mirror, mirror, on the wall, is it true I'm not small?" When I look into the mirror, I say, "Who is this old person looking back at me?"

This might be a good time to sit down and evaluate your eating habits. Are you happy with your diet? If your answer is no, it would be good to take out some paper and a pen and design a healthy eating plan. Make a decision not to go shopping for food on an empty stomach. Spend most of your time shopping around the perimeter of the grocery store. That's where most of the fruits and vegetables are kept. All the goodies, like ice cream, cereals, and snacks, and most of the carbohydrates are sold in the middle of the store.

Disturbing Discovery
I was absolutely disgusted to find out that
many brown breads are made from overrefined,
bleached white flour—then dyed brown to fool us.

Start eating meals at regular times. This includes eating a healthy breakfast—not your doughnuts and a cup of coffee. When you eat a meal, try to sit at a table and eat at a slower pace. The goal is to expand your eating time to twenty minutes rather than your usual ten minutes while you're standing or multitasking in the kitchen or another room. Why? Because after about twenty minutes, your mind triggers your body naturally and says, "You're full. Stop eating."

Serve your meals on a slightly smaller plate than you normally do. We have a tendency to eat everything on our plates. If you use a smaller plate, it will help you consume smaller amounts of food, which in turn helps you begin to lose some of the weight your mirror has been reminding you of.

I try to eat the food I put on my plate and not waste food by throwing it away. This plan becomes a little more difficult when other people put food on my plate. They stack it on with the amount they would like to eat or in an attempt to be generous to me, their guest. When this happens, I eat what I would normally eat, even if it's not everything on the plate they have given me. I do not feel the social obligation to eat everything I did not choose. You will have to set your own limits.

Too many people get uptight worrying about counting calories. You will become more at ease if you stop thinking about calories and become more concerned about feeding your cells everything they need—including vegetables and fruits on a consistent basis.

Disturbing Discovery
I was surprised to learn that many laundry detergents, softeners, and bleaches could antagonize cancer.

At the turn of the century, the average individual consumed about 10 pounds of sugar a year. Today, according to the US Department of Agriculture, the average American consumes from 150 to 170 pounds of sugar each year. That works out to be over 13 pounds of sugar a month—or more than two 5-pound sacks of sugar.

The average American drinks a little over forty-four gallons of soft drinks. A thirty-two-ounce soft drink contains over one-quarter cup of sugar. Then there is the consumption of Krispy Kreme doughnuts, Hostess Twinkies, Ding Dongs, and CupCakes, over a hundred different brands of breakfast cereals, various juice drinks, ice cream, multiple choices of snacks and candy bars, and the list goes on and on. There is no question that America has developed a sweet tooth.

Diets high in refined sugars and refined carbohydrates are dangerous because they lead to insulin resistance, which is a predictor for cancer mortality. These foods weaken the immune system. They also help to increase the inflammatory response and stimulate the release of cancer-promoting hormones. When you have inflammation, you have the generation of free radicals.

Cancer cells need, and demand, sugar for their growth. It's for this reason that many doctors recommend a low-sugar diet.

But there's a problem. If you eliminate all sugar from your diet, you will also starve healthy cells, which need sugar to provide food and energy.

"It has been estimated that about 40 percent of cancer patients do not die from cancer but from malnutrition." [4] While it is true that you need to reduce refined sugar, that does not mean you should reduce the sugar found in fruits and vegetables like tomatoes, carrots, and beets. Fruits and vegetables not only contain simple sugars but also are a valuable source of anticancer agents like carotenoids, flavonoids, cruciferous vegetables, polyphenols, and fiber, which help your body's resistance to free radical damage and cancer.

How are you doing with a sweet tooth for sugar? Don't feel as if you are alone. The majority of people love sweets. You've probably heard the comment, "Life is uncertain, so eat your desert first."

***Often a sweet tooth could be a warning
of a calcium or protein deficiency.***

If you're dealing with cancer or if you would like to work on preventing cancer, then cutting back on sugar is necessary. At this writing, I'm going on two and a half years soda-free. At least that much sugar is cut out of my life.

If you have cancer and your sugar intake is high, it can be likened to pouring gasoline on a fire in an attempt to put the fire out. You might be wise to turn off the flow of fuel and call the fire department.

Protein consists of large molecules composed of one or more long chains of amino acids. Proteins are an essential part of all living organisms.

Amino acids are organic compounds made of carbon, hydrogen, nitrogen, oxygen, or sulfur. Amino acids are the building blocks of life. They are the structural components of body tissues such as muscle, hair, collagen, and so on. Proteins also function as enzymes, hormones, and antibodies.

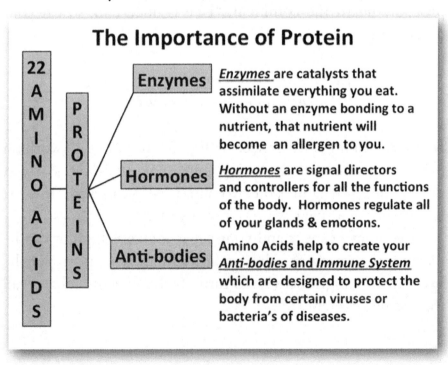

The Importance of Protein

22 AMINO ACIDS

PROTEINS

Enzymes — *Enzymes* are catalysts that assimilate everything you eat. Without an enzyme bonding to a nutrient, that nutrient will become an allergen to you.

Hormones — *Hormones* are signal directors and controllers for all the functions of the body. Hormones regulate all of your glands & emotions.

Anti-bodies — Amino Acids help to create your *Anti-bodies* and *Immune System* which are designed to protect the body from certain viruses or bacteria's of diseases.

There are two primary sources for protein: animals and plants. Plant protein is practically free from cholesterol. Plants that are high in protein are pumpkin seeds, asparagus, cauliflower, peanuts, mung seed sprouts, almonds, spinach, broccoli, and quinoa. They are high in fiber and tend to alkalize the body. There is less large-bowel cancer in people who eat high-fiber diets. Studies indicate that people who ate low-fat whole foods—mostly plant diets—"lost 2 to five pounds in 12 days; about 10 pounds after three weeks; and 16 pounds over 12 weeks." [5] Plant-based diets lower the risk for both breast cancer and heart disease. That's something to think about.

Animal protein does not have fiber and makes the body more acidic. Familiar animal proteins come from beef, chicken, turkey, fish, eggs, cheese, and milk. Research shows that cow's milk contains *casein*. It's one of the most relevant chemical *carcinogens* (cancer-causing agents) identified. Casein assists cancer cells to grow both in petri dishes and in laboratory rats. The presence or absence of casein seems to turn on or off cancer growth. There is a growing concern that cow's milk may be causing harm to those who drink it. This is setting off alarm bells in some circles and is creating an understandable concern and negative reaction in the milk-producing industry.

Cow's milk also contains bovine growth hormones, antibiotics, and pesticides. Bovine growth hormone (called rBGH) has been linked to cancer in various studies. The effect of the growth hormones, antibiotics, and pesticides on those who ingest them has yet to be determined. Quite a number of people have difficulty with dairy-related products.

In my personal experience, I used to drink a quart of milk at each meal. I also had difficulties with what is called hay fever. I constantly carried a handkerchief with me and was blowing my nose frequently. The handkerchief was usually damp with nasal discharge.

On one occasion, I was sharing with my chiropractor the difficulties I was having with sinus problems. He asked me whether I drank milk. I told him yes and the amount I was drinking. He said, "Stop drinking milk."

I followed his advice, and within about ten days, my sinus problems disappeared. I no longer carry a handkerchief with me. That was forty-three years ago.

Disturbing Discovery
I was heartbroken when I found out that many diet foods and soft drinks cause weight gain.

There are many factors that contribute toward cancer. Any single factor may not trigger the disease, but when you begin to add multiple triggers, the odds increase dramatically for cancer and other diseases.

We think there is one important word to consider when it comes to any diet and nutritional plan. It's the word *moderation*. Although I've not become a vegetarian, I'm beginning to increase my consumption of plant-based protein and decrease that of animal-based protein. Do some research, and come to your own conclusions.

The US Department of Health and Human Services lists alcoholic beverages as a known human carcinogen—a substance capable of causing cancer in living tissue. The *American Journal of Public Health* states that 3.5 percent of all cancer deaths are alcohol related. Other studies reveal that women who drink three alcoholic drinks a week have a 15 percent higher risk of breast cancer. When they drink two drinks a day, their risk factor rises by 37 percent. (6)

The drinking of alcohol—regardless of the type—has been linked to cancers of the mouth, throat, voice box, esophagus, liver, colon, rectum, pancreas, and breast. Alcohol acts as an irritant to cells. This irritation makes them susceptible to free radical damage. People who drink alcoholic beverages expose themselves to extra calories, tremors, confusion, hallucinations, seizures, increased inflammation, and hangovers.

If you're taking vitamin supplements and drinking alcohol at the same time, you're simply throwing away money and decreasing your health benefits. Alcohol impairs the body's ability to break down and absorb vitamin A, vitamin B complex, vitamin C, vitamin D, vitamin E, folate, and carotenoids. Carotenoids help to boost the immune system but lose some of their power with the use of alcohol.

Drinking with consistency over time raises the possibility of cancer damage. When you combine smoking with drinking, it raises the odds even higher. Our toast to you is that you would be much better off—and have extra money to spend—if you drank water rather than alcohol.

Each year the United States produces 530,000 tons of household hazardous waste. That's not just normal trash but waste that is hazardous to humans and the environment. The average US household generates more than twenty pounds of hazardous waste per year.

Examples of hazardous waste include the following:

adhesives	household polishes and cleaners
antifreeze	insecticides, herbicides, and
batteries	rat poisons
broken thermometers	latex and oil-based paints
cosmetics	lighter fluids
drain openers	nail polish and removers
fuel injection and carburetor	oven cleaners
cleaners	paint thinners and strippers
fungicides and wood	rat poison
preservatives	used oil and oil filters
grease and rust solvents	wood and metal cleaners

When it comes to pesticides, there are twenty thousand different products. Together they create 1.1 billion pounds of pesticides in the United States. Pesticides are the tenth-leading cause of poisoning. Under the topic of pesticides come disinfectants, fumigants, fungicides, herbicides, insecticides, repellents, and rodenticides, along with surfactants, which act as a sort of glue that holds pesticides on eatable fruits and plants.

Disturbing Discovery
I was horrified to discover that the umbilical cords
feeding our babies before they before they're born,
could have up to 144 cancer causing toxins in them.

The pesticide Roundup produced by Monsanto is particularly troubling. There is a strong link between that pesticide and cancer. Roundup has been detected in the milk of nursing mothers. You may be wise to pull up weeds rather than spray them.

When it comes to chemicals used in food, there are thirteen that have been banned by other countries but are still used in the United States. They include coloring agents *blue 1*, *blue 2*, *yellow 5*, and *yellow 6*. Other chemicals are *olestra/ Olean*, *BHA*, *BHT*, *arsenic*, and *azodicarbonamide*, which is used in making foam mats. It's also used in a number of different bakery products. Then there are the synthetic hormones *rBGH* and *rBST*, *potassium bromate*, known as brominated flour, and *brominated vegetable oil*, known as BVD. To protect your health, you should begin to read the ingredients in the foods you purchase.

It's also important to note products with *bisphenol A*. It's a *polycarbonated* plastic found in the linings of soda cans, plastic tubes of food, baby bottles, cups, and microwave bowls. Bisphenol A has a tendency to diffuse into the food products it touches.

The Fruits and Vegetables Least Contaminated by Pesticides

asparagus	eggplant	oranges
avocados	grapefruit	pineapple
bananas	kiwi	plums
blueberries	mangoes	radishes
broccoli	melons	tangerines
cabbage	mushrooms	tomatoes
cauliflower	onions	watermelons

The Fruits and Vegetables Most Contaminated by Pesticides

apples	nectarines	potatoes
celery	lettuce	raspberries
cherries	peaches	pumpkin
cucumbers	peppers	strawberries
grapes	pears	spinach
green beans	potatoes	

Disturbing Discovery

I was absolutely shocked when reading Dr. Walker's book on colon hygiene to learn that popcorn and peanut butter could be some of the unhealthiest foods in the world.

In the attempt to fight harmful bacteria, hand sanitizers were invented. Instead of using soap and water to cleanse hands, many hospitals insist on the use of antibacterial hand sanitizers. This trend has expanded to public schools, supermarkets, where many people touch the shopping cart handles, and your home for your family's use.

Your skin is the largest organ of your body. When you use hand sanitizers, oils, creams, shampoo, conditioners, body wash, and laundry detergents, the chemicals in them are absorbed into your body through your skin. Many of these products contain toxic chemicals that we unknowingly rub on our bodies. They contain *phthalates*, which are endocrine disruptors, *triclosan*, which has negative effects on hormones, and *parabens*, which mimic estrogen in the body. Parabens have been linked to breast and reproductive cancers.

The negative effective from hand sanitizers can cause an allergic reaction in some people. Hand sanitizers kill not only bad bacteria but also good bacteria that our bodies need. The killing of bacteria, which sounds good, has the detrimental effect of taking away the body's ability to develop immunity to diseases. Good old soap and water is a better answer.

Hippocrates is considered the father of medicine. He said, "Let your food be your medicine and let medicine be your food." That was written over two thousand years ago. He also suggested, "He who does not know food, how can he understand the diseases of man." It seems a shame that these concepts are not reinforced for doctors in medical schools.

When it comes to grocery store purchases, what do you think are the top twenty most popular items? They are as follows:

1. Milk	8. Coffee	15. Ice cream
2. Bread	9. Cheese	16. TV dinners
3. Eggs	10. Cereal	17. Candy
4. Chips	11. Beef	18. Yogurt
5. Soda	12. Vegetables	19. Coffee cream
6. Chicken	13. Fruit	20. Flour
7. Sugar	14. Gum	

If you're looking for vegetables that have anticancer nutrients, the following list is for you. They are listed in order as to the cancer-fighting abilities of their nutrients.

1. Garlic
2. Leeks
3. Scallions
4. Brussels sprouts
5. Savoy cabbage
6. Cabbage
7. Beets
8. Spinach
9. Kale
10. Asparagus
11. Cauliflower
12. Fiddlehead fern
13. Onions
14. Broccoli
15. Red chicory
16. Turnips
17. Eggplant
18. Red cabbage
19. Boston lettuce
20. Green beans
21. Celery
22. Potatoes
23. Bok choy
24. Fennel
25. Romaine lettuce
26. Squash
27. Carrots
28. Endive
29. Red peppers
30. Cucumbers
31. Radishes
32. Tomatoes
33. Jalapeno peppers

When you design your anticancer meals, they should include the following:

Mostly vegetables, fruits like avocados, and lentils, peas, and beans. Everything should be organic. Remove pesticides with vegetable cleaner. Cook from scratch—nothing in a box, packet, or can. Use slow cookers. Test your slow cooker with a magnet. If the magnet does not stick, it's normally not a good sign. Prepare vegetable juices and smoothies (see pages 150-152).

Grains. This includes multigrain bread, whole-grain rice, quinoa, and bulgur—organic, unbleached, and not enriched.

Fats. Recommended fats can be from avocado oil, coconut oil, grape-seed oil, olive oil, canola oil, flaxseed oil, and organic omega-3 butter. Vegetable oils (corn, soybean, sunflower, etc.), hydrogenated trans fats, conventional meat and dairy products, and nonorganic eggs contain omega-6 fatty acids. They have a tendency to cause inflammation, coagulation, and stimulation of cell growth.

On the other hand, green vegetables, flaxseed oil, canola oil, fish, and omega-3 (grass-fed) meat, dairy products, and eggs are rich in omega-3 fatty acids. They assist in the regulation of inflammation, fluidization of blood, and regulation of cell growth.

Herbs and spices. These include turmeric, mint, thyme, rosemary, and garlic.

Animal proteins are optional. They can be from fish, organic meat, omega-3 eggs, and organic dairy products, not from boxes or cans.

Random Thoughts about Diet and Eating

- In you attempt to eat healthy, try to follow the 80/20 principle. Try to eat healthy foods 80 percent of the time and trash foods 20 percent of the time. It's very doubtful that everyone can eat 100 percent healthy nutrition, especially when you eat out in restaurants.
- People who eat the most vegetables have the lowest incidence of all types of cancer.
- Keep in mind that food has the power to heal and also to harm the body. Healthy nutritional eating has the power to turn cancer complications on and off.
- It has humorously been said, "We spend millions to force people to wear safety belts and respect speed limits...so they can drive safely to the restaurants where they stuff themselves with trans fats."
- A single serving of pizza is high in calories and contains more fat from oils and cheese than an ordinary steak.
- Green tea is a wonderful cancer fighter. People who drink green tea have lower incidences of cancer. It contains numerous cancer fighters known as polyphenols. In one study, women who had breast cancer and drank three cups of green tea a day had a 50 percent reduction in relapse compared to those who drank only one cup. Men who had prostate cancer reduced their risk of

cancer progressing by 50 percent when they drank five cups of green tea a day. (7) It is best if green tea is steeped for eight to ten minutes.

- It has been shown that turmeric, a spice used in curry, inhibits the growth of colon, prostate, lung, liver, stomach, ovarian, brain, and leukemia cancers.
- It is suggested to use good salts like organic vegetable salt, Himalayan salt, sea salt, or Celtic salt.
- If you're on a budget, it's good to know that a plum contains as many antioxidants as a handful of berries. Plums cost less than berries.
- Ginger is a powerful anti-inflammatory and antioxidant.
- Dark chocolate contains polyphenols and antioxidants. The thought is yummy.
- Various mushrooms contain polysaccharides, which stimulate the immune system.
- It is best not to drink lots of water with your meals. It hampers acid breakdown of food in your stomach. It's suggested to drink little or no liquid two minutes before and thirty minutes after the meal.
- A number of studies indicate that people who eat fish at least twice a week significantly lower their risk factors for cancer.
- Bragg apple cider vinegar with the "mother" is beneficial. The "mother" consists of strands of proteins, enzymes, and friendly bacteria. It causes the vinegar to have a murky, cobweb-like appearance. The vinegar assists in killing many types of bacteria, lowers blood sugar levels, assists in fighting diabetes, helps you lose weight, lowers

cholesterol, and has protective effects against cancer. It also aids in digestion as well.

- A Chinese study found that people who ate more garlic had a 60 percent reduction in stomach cancer [8]

Disturbing Discovery
I was startled to discover that antifreeze (propylene glycol) is used in some ice creams. It helps to stabilize the temperature and keep the ice cream from becoming too hard for the customer to scoop out of the container.

Cancer is a genetic disease. What does that mean? It means that the genes within our individual cells (our DNA) become damaged. The damage is caused primarily by free radicals, as mentioned in chapter 1.

Confusion arises when you hear the word *genetic* and think it means that cancer is inherited from your family of origin. Very little of any type of cancer is passed down from our relatives. Only 5–10 percent of all cancers are hereditary.

Many women fear they will get breast cancer because someone in their families had breast cancer. Unfortunately, because of this fear, there are many who have their breasts removed when it's not necessary.

You may think that because someone in your family has cancer, you will also get it. Yes, it could happen, but it's rare. However, you may have indeed inherited something that is not a disease. You may have inherited a pattern or lifestyle of eating cancer-producing foods and food additives.

If you grew up eating pizza, drinking soda, enjoying lots of beef, eating few vegetables, and loading up with pastries and ice cream, yes, you inherited an unhealthy lifestyle from your family. It's not a cancer-producing gene. It's a cancer-producing lifestyle. That's what most people inherit. How healthy of an eating pattern did your family of origin establish for you?

> *The last time I had a hot meal was*
> *when a candle fell in my TV dinner.*

Late October 2008, I was diagnosed with aggressive stage 4 breast cancer. There was noticeable activity in my liver and two-plus liters of fluid between the lining of my right lung and chest wall. The fluid was removed and tested. Full-body scans were done to help in determining my treatment plan. Within three weeks I began chemotherapy that would take me into April 2009. The chemo would shrink my tumor to the degree that surgery would have the most successful outcome.

In February 2009, my first grandchild was born, and I was strong enough to be present at her birth! What a joy this was in the midst of everything else going on.

Chemo ended on a Friday, leaving me fatigued but otherwise doing well. Lab work showed tumor markers coming down, which was another promising sign, but there was an achiness in the thigh of my left leg. This was not particularly unusual, since for years I had been seeing a chiropractor off and on owing to an earlier injury. For the next week, some days were better than others, but I was happy to be at work, something I enjoyed.

Thursday of the week following the end of chemo, I was on my feet almost all day and was definitely tired. Going to bed, I slept hard, but I woke refreshed. As I moved to sit up on the edge of the bed, my leg began to hurt. I stood and hobbled to the restroom but asked my husband for support to make it back to the bedroom. I sat in the chair next to the bed and began to pray. I decided to call my oncologist and tell her about my leg. I knew I couldn't go to work. She told me to meet her at the hospital emergency room and she would schedule an x-ray to see what was going on.

The next hour or so was nothing short of chaos and excruciating pain as I attempted to leave for the hospital. Our bedroom was upstairs, and I could barely walk and now could barely move. Let me just say my ride to the hospital was an unique and difficult experience in the back of a paramedic ambulance!

Arriving at the hospital, I was greeted by my doctor and quickly taken to x-ray, and within an hour, I had the results—a broken left femur! Really?

I received lots of questions from the doctors and staff.

"Did you fall?"

"What have you been doing?"

"No" and "Nothing unusual" were my answers. Surgery was scheduled for the following morning. Doctors expected to find bone cancer, soft and spongy bone. When they opened me up, the bone was perfect, strong and healthy, but broken. How and why, I don't know, but I believe God healed it!

With my mastectomy pending, recovery needed to be four weeks between surgeries, and that was pushing it. I was doing a lot of praying during this time, asking the Lord to strengthen my body in preparation for the surgery still to come. He answered my prayers, and I was feeling ready.

The time couldn't have come quick enough for my breast surgeons, who were waiting to do the surgery mid-May 2009. That surgery left me with another eight to ten weeks of recovery before

I began my radiation treatment in August 2009. Treatments (thirty-five to be exact) would clear the possibility of any remaining cancer left in the margins from surgery. Radiation finished up in October, and the two months leading up to Christmas was a wonderful time to rest and enjoy the holidays and family time.

I continued seeing my oncologist every three months, in addition to continuing the standard labs and scans that follow chemotherapy. Results were improving.

Suddenly, in April 2010, I had a facial seizure. Following two days in the ICU, I had an MRI, which determined I had a grape-sized brain tumor.

My oncologist met with a team of doctors to discuss the course of treatment I should receive. They felt I was a prime candidate for CyberKnife, a new state-of-the-art robotic administration of radiation.

When released from the hospital, I met with the doctor who would oversee this treatment. Preparation was begun, and within days the CyberKnife was administered. The Lord again blessed me with excellent care and results. The DNA of the tumor was destroyed, and only the scar tissue remained, which would dissipate over time, and it did.

Following this, I was told by the doctor to rest and cut my activity level in half for the next three to four months to allow my body time to fully recover from all it had been through. This seemed doable since I would also be going through occupational and physical therapy for my temporary speech difficulties and the weakness that occurred in my right side owing to the seizure. With God's miraculous care and healing, these challenges were soon resolved.

Unfortunately, I guess I did too good a job of resting, because the next month, in May, I got a DVT (blood clot) in my right leg. I had surgery to place a filter in the main artery that would block the clot from traveling to my heart and lungs. I was told to elevate my leg as much as possible, not to sit for long periods, and to rest. I was put on Coumadin and was told I would probably be on it for the rest of my life.

What? Are you kidding me? Not when I found out it was rat poison! I said, "We'll see." I was going to do my best to get off it ASAP!

During this time, in June 2010, my daughter Heather and I began seeing a nutritionist, and I started taking whole food supplements. I wanted to overcome my fatigue and chemo brain/fog and help my body battle back from all I had been through, but after a few months, I didn't feel much different. I was also dealing with elevated vitamin K levels while on the Coumadin owing to my consumption of raw fruits and vegetables and some whole food supplements. This kept the doctors in the clinic on their toes to continually adjust my dosage with weekly blood tests.

In October 2010, by divine appointment, my son Johnny introduced me to Louis and LaVerne Smith at Hume Lake Christian Camps, where the three of them had met a few months before. My husband and I spent three days with Louis and his wife going over my health challenges, my desire for changes, the supplements I was currently taking, and the benefits of juicing and a healthy diet.

It was life changing! We learned new things about nutrition, whole food supplements based in nature and backed by science, organics, washing produce to remove pesticides, and so much more! At the conclusion of the three days, we purchased supplements Louis told us about. I was excited to try them, and we planned to meet again in two weeks to follow up and compare the supplements I had been taking before with the new ones from Louis.

The two weeks quickly passed; it was now November 2010, and I was beginning to feel less fatigued. There were definitely some changes taking place. When Louis and I met, we compared supplements. In doing so, I learned that although the ones I had been taking were made from whole foods, they were isolates and were not grouped together as they are found in nature.

For example, I had been taking calcium and magnesium independently. This is not how they are found in nature. They should be together in a 2:1 ratio for proper absorption in the body. Several other supplements were troublesome for the same reasons. After going through all of them, I was able to lessen the number of supplements and save money taking better-quality ones.

As my body continued to respond to the changes in supplements, I was ready to take the whole regime to battle against cancer and all I had dealt with from the months of treatment. I was ready to tackle the chemo brain, the fatigue, the muscle atrophy, and weak bones, detox from the chemotherapy and radiation, and renew my strength.

I wanted to be healthy again and fully live the second chance I had been given. Time and time again, when friends and family saw the change in me, they started asking questions, and soon many wanted what we had done. Not because they were all fighting cancer, but they had fatigue, a general lack of vitality, or a need for weight loss.

The whole food supplements I was taking are second to none! They have had a tremendous impact on my health. Aside from my being off all medication, my chemo brain is gone; fatigue is now only a by-product of lack of sleep and busy schedules. My muscle atrophy is a thing of the past; my labs are all in the normal range. I feel better today than I did precancer. I've even participated in six 5Ks with my daughter Haleigh, something I never thought would be possible.

Fast-forward to just before Christmas 2013. My oncologist told me my recovery was remarkable and not at all what was expected when I was first diagnosed in 2008. She said the board of doctors reviewing my case were calling me their "poster child" and wanted to reopen my case to look at what was different about me in comparison to other cases similar to mine. In addition, she gave me the greatest Christmas present I've ever received, saying that typically her metastatic patients with my aggressive stage 4 breast cancer must wait seven to ten years, but with my case, five years from diagnosis, she was confident in saying that I WAS IN REMISSION!

She warned me to not change a thing I was doing, noting that my emphasis on nutrition and supplementation and my faith, family support, and positive attitude held great significance. I couldn't agree more.

I know that my divine appointment in 2010 was the beginning of a new life, a new story, and a new me. In the past six and a half years, the supplements I have taken have touched my life in ways I never expected. I am so thankful to the Lord for allowing my son to introduce me to Louis and LaVerne Smith so my husband and I could learn about living a healthy lifestyle. I am forever indebted.

Disturbing Discovery
*It was unbelievable to learn that cancer thrives
on sugar—yet in my cancer specialist's reception
room for cancer patients, there were
cookies and candy for them to eat.*

C hronic disease has become a worldwide health crisis. In 1912, heart disease was nearly nonexistent. Today heart disease is the number-one killer. Strokes are on the increase.

Cancer is on the rise. One hundred years ago, only 3 percent of Americans died from cancer. Today, 50 percent of Americans encounter some type of cancer. Breast cancer is one of the most talked-about killers. Over two hundred thousand men a year are diagnosed with prostate cancer.

The leading cause of respiratory disease is cigarette smoking. Over twelve million people suffer from this disorder. From 1980 to 2010, diabetes increased by 176 percent. It's now the seventh-leading cause of death in the United States.

Everyone is talking about health. Television, the Internet, newspapers, magazines, and books are filled with health tips and advice for losing weight. The National Center for Health Statistics estimated that 66.7 percent of Americans are overweight or obese. Childhood obesity is increasing at an alarming rate.

Over one million Americans live with Parkinson's. It's estimated that 1.1 percent of people in the United States have the disease and are not aware of it. Alzheimer's and dementia now affect over fifteen million Americans to some degree.

Osteoporosis is a growing concern among women. It's estimated that there will be 1.5 million fractures this year owing to this disease. Over fifty million people have some form of arthritis, gout, lupus, or fibromyalgia. Asthma is on the rise, along with ADHD, among children.

Disorder, disease, and disability are affecting millions. What in the world is going on? As we consider chronic disease, the cause and the cure are the same: diet and lifestyle. World health leaders all agree that there are three major health issues. They are unhealthy diet, lack of exercise, and cigarette smoking.

How are we to deal with all these health issues? It must be remembered that treatment for the body comes from without. Doctors usually address symptoms. Healing for the body, however, comes from within. God has designed the human body with the ability to heal itself if given the proper nourishment and protection from unwanted toxins.

Getting the proper nourishment for the body has become more and more of a challenge. Many farms have overutilized soils, which have become depleted of nourishment. In 1948, the mineral content of spinach was 150 milligrams per bowl. By 1998, the mineral content of spinach had dropped to 2 milligrams per bowl.

Along with soil depletion has come an increase in hybridizing, genetically modified organisms (GMOs), and pasteurization of fruit and vegetable juices. It is becoming increasingly more difficult to remove oil-based sprays from fruits and vegetables. Added to these factors are the advanced use of pesticides and systemics and the storing of fresh foods for months. All these factors lead to nutrient reduction or damage.

More confusion continues with white sugar, which is really bleached brown sugar. White bread is bleached from yellowish wheat flour. Then the white flour is colored brown and sold as wheat bread. Items like chicken nuggets, hotdogs, bologna, pepperoni, salami, and jerky are made from mechanically separated meats, or MSMs. Then the meats are put into mechanical forms that produce exact duplicates of chicken breasts and other shapes depending on the product desired.

More and more people are realizing they're not getting all the proper nutrients they need from fast foods, processed foods, and whole foods grown with GMOs and covered with pesticides or filled with systemic pesticides.

Everyone has a busy schedule. We're all faced with the depletion of food nutrients. We're all exposed to a vast amount of toxins. Because of this, more and more people are turning to supplements to fill the nutritional gaps in their diets.

More than half of all adult Americans take at least one dietary supplement. Parents are also concerned for the health of their children and are providing vitamins for them to take. That's good news. But there is also bad news. Most of the vitamin, mineral, and protein supplements that adults and children are taking are made from synthetics rather than human whole food.

Disturbing Discovery
It was unbelievable to me to learn that the US Food and Drug Administration allows the sale of certain

*supplements that contain ingredients that can
actually harm us instead of healing us.*

The major producer and exporter of vitamin, mineral, and protein supplements and drugs is China. China controls 90 percent of the raw-ingredient market for supplementation. It's also estimated that 90 percent of vitamin C is produced in China.

In an attempt to keep this discussion simple, we will say there are basically two types of nutrients: natural, whole food nutrients and artificial or synthetic nutrients. Natural, whole food nutrients come from living plants and animals that have carbon molecules. Artificial or synthetic nutrients are created from nonliving and inert synthetic chemicals.

Why would manufacturers use synthetic chemicals rather than natural whole foods from the human food chain? The answer is simple: they are easier and cheaper to obtain. It's more costly to grow, harvest, and process real plant and animal nutrients. These synthetics are designed to look and taste like the real thing, but they're not.

You can't fool your body. God created your immune system, which identifies those synthetics as toxins and not as real food. Now your body has to attempt to keep you healthy by getting rid of these foreign (synthetic) substances. The battle is now on.

You put these synthetics into your body with the assumption that they will make you healthy. However, they are doing just the opposite. They are helping you become ill. The synthetics have no bioavailability to give your body what it needs to survive. No wonder there is an increase of health issues in our country.

Those who produce synthetic supplements will argue that synthetics are as good as human-food-chain supplements. But what is produced in the laboratory cannot compare with what God has created. Scientists can chemically reproduce seawater that looks like seawater, tastes like seawater, and has all the chemical properties of seawater. But there is one problem. Put a fish in this synthetic seawater, and see what happens. The fish will die.

There is a nutrient called beta carotene. It's found in a number of different vegetables. It's essential for health in the human body. Scientists have created a synthetic beta carotene that comes from acetylene gas.

There is a nutrient called d-alpha tocopherol. It's one of the eight E vitamins and is an essential whole food and good for your health. The same synthetic nutrient is called dl-alpha tocopherol. It is found in almost every name-brand vitamin E on the market, and you can tell it is synthetic by the "dl" before the "alpha." The "d" before the "alpha" is short for *dextro*, which means "right." Natural d-alpha tocopherol has a right-leaning molecule when exposed to light. The "dl" means there is a split and the vitamin E is composed of a right-leaning molecule and a left-leaning (*levo*) molecule, which the body has a difficult time recognizing and proceeds to eliminate.

If you want to identify synthetic chemicals in your supplements, look for the following names. They will identify a few of the ingredients that are *not* healthy for your body.

acetate
aminobenzoic acid
ascorbate
ascorbic acid
aspartate
calciferol
calcium d-
pantothenate
carbonate
choline bitartrate
chloride
citrate
dl-alpha tocopherol
d-biotin
disulfide
dibasic phosphate

gluconate
glycerophosphate
hydrochloride
hydroxyyapatitehydro
xyapatite
iodide,
irradiated ergosteral
lactate
malate
menadione
methionine
mononitrate
niacin
orotate
oxide,
palmiatepalmitate

phytonadione
picolinate
pteroylglutamic
acid
pyridoxine
hydrochloride
pyrophosphate
riboflavin
silicon dioxide
stearate
succinate
thiamine
hydrochloride
thiamine
mononitrate
tribasic phosphate

The US National Cancer Institute found that men taking more than one synthetic vitamin a day might increase their risk of prostate cancer by 32 percent and nearly double their risk of fatality. [9]

In 2007, a report in the *Journal of the American Medical Association* showed that those taking synthetic antioxidants (i.e., beta carotene) increased their risk of dying by up to 16 percent. [10]

Dr. Lester Packer says that if you take synthetic vitamin E instead of natural vitamin E, it will have an immediate loss of 36 percent in nutritional value. [11]

Dr. Arthur Furst says that synthetic amino acids are identified by our enzymes and discarded as 100 percent waste from the body.

Dr. Linus Palings says that there is about a 50 percent loss of absorption between synthetic ascorbic acid and organic natural vitamin C.

Dr. Rois says that no one knows why a whole food is more beneficial, but the theory is that God produces a perfect balance that can't be reproduced in a laboratory.

Not only is it important to look for natural, organic, whole food supplements, but it is also good to consider the following when selecting vitamin, mineral, and protein products.

- How long has the company been in business?
- Does the Food and Drug Administration license its facility?
- Does the company have any lawsuits or fraud cases filed against it?
- Where does it get ingredients for supplements? Are the ingredients produced in the United States or out of country?
- Does the company manufacture its own products? Does it have its own dedicated facility and equipment for doing this? Or is it simply a distributor for other manufacturers?
- Are the products made from organic, natural whole foods?
- Are the products free from synthetics, dyes, pesticides, systemics, and GMOs?
- Does the company employ its own staff of scientists?
- Has the company presented scientific research papers in publications like the *New England Journal of Medicine*,

Journal of the American College of Nutrition, International Journal of Toxicology, or *American Journal of Clinical Nutrition?*

- Does the company seem to follow health fads, or is it based more on scientific research?
- Does the company have any "seal of approval" by an outside agency that evaluates the accuracy of the products and what they contain?
- Does its vitamin E products contain all eight vitamin Es (four tocopherols and four tocotrienols)? Does its vitamin E say "d-alpha-tocopherol" and not "dl-alpha-tocopherol"?
- Do its products contain both *lipids* and *sterols?*

Disturbing Discovery
It's incredible to me that it's legal to sell food that contain toxins, colorants, preservatives, and flavorings that can antagonize cancer.

- Are some of its products *chelated* (the process of combining organic compounds)?
- Does its *calcium* contain two parts calcium and one part magnesium along with 1,000 IU for vitamin D_3?
- Is its *salmon oil* cold pressed rather than heated? Does it contain all eight known oils from the fish family? Has its salmon oil been tested for at least two hundred toxins, like mercury and lead?
- Does its *acidophilus* contain a broad spectrum of the five types of beneficial lactic acid–producing bacteria:

Lactobacillus acidophilus, Lactobacillus bulgaricus, Lactobacillus casei, Bifidobacterium bifidum, and *Streptococcus thermophiles?*

- Is its *calcium* and *magnesium* chelated?
- Do its *carotenoids* contain all fifteen whole food families?
- Is its *CoQ10* extracted from whole food fruits and vegetables?
- Does its *fiber* provide all five types of dietary fiber necessary for good health, including cellulose, hemicellulose, gum, lignin, and pectin?
- Do its *flavonoids* contain flavonoids representative of all flavonoid classes: flavones, flavonols, flavanones, anthocyanins, and catechins as they naturally occur in human-food-chain fruits and vegetables?
- Does its *garlic with allium* include not only allicin but also other bioactive compounds (for example, oil-soluble substances from fresh garlic and onion)? Does its garlic with allium have an enteric coating to maximize the product's stability and absorption and insure the formation of active allicin in the intestines?
- Does its *glucosamine* provide 1,500 milligrams of glucosamine, the therapeutic dose shown in studies to reduce pain and stiffness? Does it come from glucosamine hydrochloride, which is sulfite-free and easy to digest?
- Does its *iron* contain double amino acid chelates to support more efficient iron absorption, and is it chelated?
- Does its *lecithin* contain active phospholipids choline (175 milligrams) and inositol (100 milligrams), the two most important dietary contributors of lipotropic factors involved in nerve transmission?

- Does its *protein powder* contain all twenty-two amino acids necessary for cell health? Does its protein powder contain fiber? Is it free from artificial sweeteners, colors, and flavors? Is it free from saturated fats, preservatives, GMOs, gluten, high-fructose corn syrup, and hydrogenated fats / trans fats, and is it 90 percent lactose-free? Protein should also be fermented, predigested, or *protoguarded* (a process to protect amino acids and maximize nutritional value) to protect your kidneys and to increase utilization.

The above questions are designed to assist you in finding trusted natural, organic, whole food manufacturers.

You can purchase supplements at a supermarket, drug store, or health food store or directly from the manufacturer on the Internet. Supermarkets and drug stores carry a great deal of popular name-brand synthetic vitamins, minerals, and protein supplements. They very seldom stock natural, organic, whole food supplements. Whole food products usually cost a little more because it is more expensive to produce quality products rather than the cheaper synthetics.

Health food stores carry a large variety of products. Most likely over half of their supplements contain synthetics. They do, however, also carry whole food products. The caution here is that the whole foods (and the synthetics) are often broken down into isolates. Let me give you an example of an isolate. I'm sure that you have heard of the vitamin B complex. The complex is made up of all the B vitamins. An isolate is when you single out one of the Bs, like vitamin B_{12}. Many people take only isolates.

We personally prefer to take the entire B complex because that's the way it comes in nature. Nature does not create isolates; scientists do. When you combine all the Bs together, they work in synergy together. Each person has to come to his or her own conclusion, accompanied by the advice of a medical professional.

- Keep in mind that although whole food supplements are beneficial, the best nutrition comes from eating with your fork and spoon. Supplements help fill nutritional gaps, but it's still important to eat real food. Think about it. We have been eating real food for thousands of years. Refer to the foods mentioned under the "Diet" section.
- Vitamin C is a very important because cancer cells gobble it up. It's very similar in structure to sugar, which cancer cells love. Vitamin C is an antioxidant that helps reduce kidney and other cancers while protecting healthy tissue from the damaging effects of chemotherapy and radiation.
- Pineapple contains an element called *bromelain*. Not only is it a pain reducer, but also it helps dissolve the coating on cancer cells so T cells can identify them and destroy them.
- A deficiency in vitamin A increases the risk of lung cancer. It has been shown to slow down and reverse some forms of cancer. In one study it reduced the damage from mouth cancer by 96 percent [12]
- Individuals with an intake of vitamin E had a 40 percent reduction in their risk for colon cancer. [13]
- Vitamin D inhibits the growth of breast cancer.

- Carotenoids are plant pigments responsible for bright red, yellow, and orange hues in many fruits and vegetables. Foods containing carotenoids will boost the immune system by 37 percent in about twenty days.

Disturbing Discovery
I was shocked to learn that certain skin creams and sunscreens can antagonize cancer.

Synergy is the action of two or more agents or forces in such a way that their combined effect is greater than the sum of their individual efforts. Author Dave Ramsey, in his book entitled *Entreleadership*, gives an example of synergy using horses.

> One of the largest, strongest horses in the world is the Belgian draft horse. Competitions are held to see which horse can pull the most and one Belgian can pull 8,000 pounds. The weird thing is if you put two Belgian horses in the harness who are strangers to each other, together they can pull 20,000–24,000 pounds. Two can pull not twice as much as one but three times as much as one. This example represents the power of synergy. However, if the two horses are raised and trained together they learn to pull and think as one. The trained, and therefore unified, pair can pull 30,000–32,000 pounds, almost four times as much as a single horse.

When it comes to nutrition, each individual nutrient has an important effect on the body. However, when you combine nutrients together, there's a synergy that takes place. It increases the positive benefits received more than if the nutrients were alone.

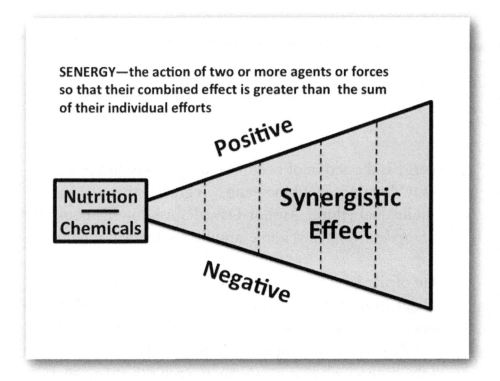

SENERGY—the action of two or more agents or forces so that their combined effect is greater than the sum of their individual efforts

Positive

Nutrition
——
Chemicals

Synergistic Effect

Negative

But synergy can also have a compound negative effect. In one study, animals were fed a human food additive, and there were no adverse results. When fed a second, different food additive, the animals began balding, had diarrhea, and lost weight. When a third food additive was added, the animals died within two weeks. [14]

A good example of negative synergy can be seen in humans when you combine toxic substances and unhealthy lifestyles together. Let's take smoking, alcohol, a poor diet, lack of exercise, increased stress, and obesity. When combined together, these six negative factors increase the odds of your getting cancer dramatically. As you decrease any of the above, the incidences of cancer also decrease.

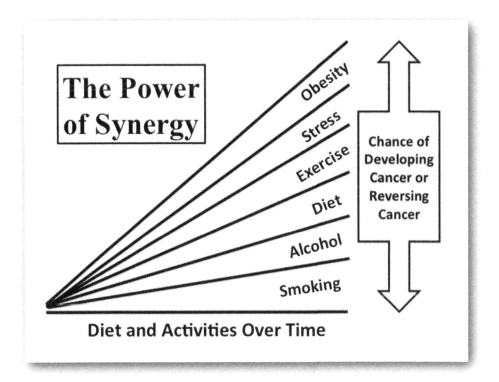

In a sense, you could liken the combination vitamins, minerals, and proteins to concrete. How do you make concrete? You start with some sand. Is sand a good foundation by itself? Then you add some crushed or rounded rock. Is crushed or rounded rock by itself a good foundation? Next you put in some cement powder. Is cement powder by itself a good foundation? Finally, you add some water. Is water by itself a good foundation?

Making a firm foundation of concrete happens only when the individual ingredients come together in synergy to create something they could not do individually by themselves. This is, in effect, what needs to happen when we eat the various nutrients on the food pyramid. They give you a solid foundation of good health and well-being.

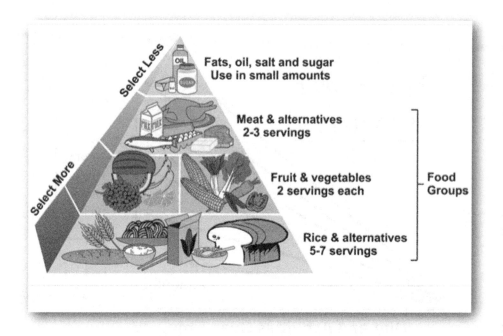

*Health is the thing that makes you feel that now is
the best time of the year.*
—Franklin Pierce Adams

The term *pH* represents the potential of hydrogen level in your blood. When a doctor measures your pH level, he or she is attempting to determine the balance between acid and alkaline in your blood. Why is this important? Because acidic blood is related to almost every disease in some way.

Listed below is an extensive but not exhaustive list of diseases and disorders that researchers have linked to acidity in the blood. If your doctor indicates you might have any of the possible disorders, ask him or her to test your blood pH to determine whether your body is acidic. Changing your body from acidic to alkaline will assist your immune system in fighting cancer.

allergies
ALS or Lou Gehrig's
Alzheimer's disease
arteriosclerosis
arthritis
bone fractures
bronchitis
cancer
candidiasis
cardiovascular disease
chronic fatigue
syndrome

chronic infections
dementia
depression
diabetes
fibromyalgia
heart attacks
high blood pressure
high cholesterol
hormonal imbalances
immune deficiencies
insulin insensitivity
kidney disease

multiple sclerosis
muscular dystrophy
osteoporosis
Parkinson's disease
premature aging
premature hair
graying
prostate problems
senility
sinusitis
stroke
weight problems

Disturbing Discovery
I was shocked to learn that some tea bags contain cancer-causing substances.

The answer to good health does not lie in the hands of doctors or large pharmaceutical companies. They treat only symptoms. Good health begins with God's creation of the foods you eat and the type of water you drink. It has been said that food is the best medicine you can take.

However, there is a problem. Pesticides, antibiotics, synthetic hormones, unnatural chemicals, genetic modifications, biochemical alterations, depletion of soils, and other factors have damaged our food chain. There are over eighty thousand industrial chemicals being used in our country. It's almost impossible not to be exposed to many of them in our daily lives.

It has been estimated that there are over three thousand additives and preservatives that have been inserted into our food-supply system. These additives come in the form of coloring agents, artificial flavors, flavor enhancers, chemically altered fats and sugars, stabilizers, conditioners, thickeners, texturizers, synthetic fillers, bleaching agents, ripening gases, waxes, petroleum products, heavy metals, and preservatives. It's also been estimated that the average person consumes about 124 pounds of food chemicals each year. Yum, yum. The body then has to deal with these foreign and indigestible substances. It's not surprising that a person's immune system is on constant overload.

Many of the foods we eat tend to be acidic rather than alkaline. What makes these types of foods so attractive? The answer can be found in one word: *sugar*. You'll remember that at the turn of the century, our great-grandparents consumed about 10 pounds of sugar a year. Today the average person consumes around 150 to 170 pounds of refined sugar inserted into various food products. This does not even include artificial sweeteners like aspartame, saccharin, and other products the body has to eliminate.

Sugar has a tendency to block our immune response for four to six hours. This is not helpful if we are fighting viruses, bacteria, and other pathogens. There is a strong tie between sugar and cancer, hormonal disruptions, arthritis, osteoporosis, cataracts, and other degenerative diseases. Added to the sugar are the sixty chemicals used in the refining process. These include bleaches and deodorizers.

The foods you choose to eat determine your body's pH balance. If you eat a lot of sweets, meat, dairy products, trans fats, white flour, fried foods, and chemical additives, your system will become acidic. You can test your pH by purchasing a tube of test strips from your pharmacy.

Acid							Neutral			Alkaline			
1	2	3	4	5	6	7	8	9	10	11	12	13	14

7.356

For example, let's look at one of our favorite drinks, carbonated soda beverages. It is estimated that the average person consumes fifty-two gallons of highly acidic soda a year. Coco-Cola measures 2.52 on the pH scale. Research suggests that it takes 32 glasses of water with a pH reading of 7.0 to neutralize one glass of soda, diet or otherwise. [15] How much soda do you drink?

Not only does the average person eat foods that are very acidic, but we usually do not drink enough water with a pH of at least 7.0. It has been estimated that 75 percent of the world's population is chronically dehydrated. It has been suggested that 45–80 percent of colon cancer, breast cancer, bladder cancer, joint pain, and back pain can be reduced by drinking eight to nine glasses of water a day.

If you have strong cravings for acid-forming junk food, it's usually your body's signal that you are dehydrated. Eating those types of food will not hydrate you, and you'll put on weight. Instead, drink an eight-ounce glass of water, which will help with hydration and also decrease your desire for junk foods. Now that's a win-win situation.

Signs of being acidic can include strong-smelling urine, arthritis, taking a lot of aspirin (acetylsalicylic acid), gout, lupus, and other disorders previously mentioned. Being overweight or underweight can also be a sign of high acid levels. The depletion of calcium and magnesium is another sign of too much acid in the body. Any type of cancer in the body is usually an indication that the body is highly acidic. Cancer and other disorders have difficulty surviving and spreading if the body is alkaline.

Foods high in acid include milk and dairy products, beef and pork, white potatoes, canned fruits, white flower, refined sugar, alcohol, fruit juices, and items like table salt, ketchup, mayonnaise, mustard, yeast, malt, and margarine. Although we cannot eliminate all these items, we can reduce our intake of them.

To help kick the acid habit, we can reduce our intake of sugar and artificial sweeteners, fried foods, goodies like cake, doughnuts, and pies, soda drinks, fast-food burgers and fries, onion rings, tacos, pizza, chips, Slurpees, alcohol, over-the-counter medications, boxed cereals, and microwaveable meals. Wow! There goes most of our nutrition.

You can also add fresh lemon juice (a half a lemon) to your eight-ounce glass of water. That will help to balance your pH level. If you don't have a lemon available, you can add one-quarter of a spoon of baking soda to your glass of water. It will do the same thing. However, it doesn't taste quite as good as lemon.

Clinical nutritionist Jim McAfee has compiled a short list of interesting facts about water and its importance in our lives.

- Seventy-five percent of Americans are chronically dehydrated (this likely applies to half the world population).
- In 37 percent of Americans, the thirst mechanism is so weak that it is often mistaken for hunger.
- Even mild dehydration will slow down one's metabolism as much as 3 percent.
- One glass of water shut down midnight hunger pangs for almost 100 percent of dieters studied in a University of Washington study.
- Lack of water is the number-one trigger of daytime fatigue.
- Preliminary research indicates that eight to ten glasses of water a day could significantly ease back and joint pain for up to 80 percent of sufferers.
- A mere 2 percent drop in body water can trigger fuzzy short-term memory, trouble with basic math, and difficulty focusing on a computer screen or a printed page.
- Drinking five glasses of water daily decreases the risk of colon cancer by 45 percent; plus it can slash the risk of breast cancer by 79 percent, and you are 50 percent less likely to develop bladder cancer.

Drinking an adequate amount of water is critical to support optimal cellular and tissue function. The survival rule of thumb suggests that you can live three weeks without food, three days without water, three hours without shelter in bad weather, and three minutes without oxygen. Our bodies consist primarily of water in the following percentages:

blood: 83 percent
bones: 22 percent
brain: 74 percent
connective tissue: 60 percent

fat: 20 percent
kidneys: 83 percent
liver: 86 percent
muscles: 76 percent
skin: 70 percent

This is not new information. We've all heard about eating well-balanced meals and drinking healthy water. The question is, how many people eat well-balanced meals and drink enough healthy water? How many people attempt to balance their pH levels? In a USDA study of twenty thousand people, how many of those studied do you think ate well-balanced meals and received their daily requirements for vitamins, minerals, and protein? [16] The answer is *no one.*

That's why in our busy schedules it's important to consider taking nutritional supplements to fill in the gaps in our daily diets. How important is health to you? Someone said that our first wealth is health. Are you really feeling healthy? Why not? Are you eating correctly? Why not? Are you experiencing health issues? Are you tired of being sick?

You see, we change our habits only when we hurt enough. Which is more important to you: eating sweets and being dehydrated, or eating healthy and drinking healthy water? You can manage your eating and pH balance. Treatment for the body comes from the outside. Healing for the body comes from the inside. The choice is yours. What do you want to do?

Health is the thing that makes you feel that
now is the best time of the year.
—Franklin Pierce Adams

Burgie Layman's Story

In September 2014 I was diagnosed with stage 1 multiple myeloma cancer. At the time I had lesions in the back of my pelvic bone. My oncologist started my treatment with Velcade shots in the stomach, twenty-five milligrams of Revlimid, forty milligrams of dexamethasone, and Zometa, which was injected intravenously.

My IGG count was around 4,300 at the time of the diagnosis. That's the measurement of the protein in the blood. The range, according to the chart, should be 700–1,600. After I was on the treatment program for approximately three months, it went down to 1,133.

The treatment knocked me off my feet with the side effects from extreme constipation to extreme diarrhea. It put me in the hospital with double pneumonia, and my potassium went down to 2; the low end of the range is 3.5. In the hospital I was having one bag of potassium after another intravenously.

I lost sixty-five pounds, could not take a shower on my own, and had to use a wheelchair when going out. I did not drive for five months. I was just wasting away. While on treatment I did not take any supplements, as per the doctor's request.

During the sixteen months after returning home from the hospital, I did not receive any chemotherapy treatments. I did, however, start back up with a regime of megadoses of whole food supplements. My wife continued juicing for me every day.

During this time my IGG count fluctuated up and down but stayed in the normal range.

After sixteen months I had to start treatment again, but not with the Velcade shots and with a lower dose of Revlimid and the dexamethasone along with the Zometa intravenously once a month.

This type of cancer is incurable and can only be put in remission. After starting treatment again, I stayed on my regime of supplements and juicing daily. In my opinion the most important supplements were the lipids and sterols, salmon oil, carotenoids, and vitamins and minerals. They were an important part in helping keep my immune system up so it could fight the cancer.

I stay away from sugar, high-fructose corn syrup, processed foods, and GMOs. I now read a lot of labels to ensure that the contents are made from whole foods and not synthetics. My remission can be attributed to supplements, lifestyle changes, and removing toxins from my life.

The medical industry had given up with me and sent me home to die. That's when I decided I wanted to live. I became a health fanatic. My incredible wife helped and empowered me to create the right environment for my body to heal itself.

Our bodies contain about sixty thousand miles of blood vessels. Smaller blood vessels are called capillaries. We have about nineteen billion capillaries. Blood vessels and capillaries bring oxygen and nutrition to all our cells.

Angiogenesis is a very complex process whereby our bodies can create or sprout new blood vessels from old blood vessels. This process naturally occurs in growth and development after the embryo stage. Once a young person reaches a certain growth period, angiogenesis tapers off and discontinues—except in the case of growth within a woman's uterus, the development of the placenta, when there has been a wound to the body that needs repair, or growth that happens as a result of disease.

When cells become damaged because of free radicals, infection, or inflammation, they reproduce themselves as another damaged cell. Damaged cells then form small clusters of cancerous cells about the size of the round ball in a ballpoint pen. They form a small microtumor. At this point the small clusters of cancer cells are harmless. Why are they harmless? Because they do not have blood vessels bringing them oxygen and nourishment so they can grow.

By the time women reach fifty years of age, 40 percent of them will have microtumors in their breasts. The same is true for men in that by the time they are fifty to sixty years of age, 50 percent of them will have microtumors in their prostate. By the time both men and women reach their seventies, they will have microtumors in their thyroids.

It's important to understand how the microtumors of cancer begin to grow and become dangerous and life threatening. The small cluster of cancerous cells has the ability to secrete blood vessel growth factors like *VEGF* and *bFGF*. There are at least twenty different known angiogenic growth factors. These factors stimulate and encourage blood vessels to move toward the cancerous cluster. Capillaries then grow toward the cluster and eventually begin feeding the cluster. Its favorite food is sugar. As the cluster begins to grow, the need for more capillaries increases.

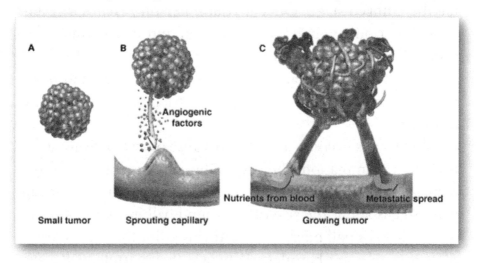

In the diagram above, A represents the small harmless tumor. Next is B, which illustrates the *angiogenic factors* that stimulate the capillary to begin to sprout and move toward the cluster. C symbolizes nutrients from the blood feeding the cluster on the left side. On the right side, it indicates the pathway from the cluster back to the bloodstream. This is how the cluster metastasizes and passes cancerous cells to other parts of the body. That's the bad news.

The process of angiogenesis is not limited to cancer. It's involved in about seventy other diseases and disorders. They include the following:

Alzheimer's	chronic wounds	endometriosis
arthritis	coronary heart	erectile dysfunction
cancer	disease	hair loss
macular degeneration	obesity	rosacea
multiple sclerosis	psoriasis	stroke
nerve damage		

Now for the good news! Cutting-edge research has discovered about three hundred *antiangiogenic* inhibitors, which stop or slow down the growth of blood vessels in the cancerous clusters. There are a number of drugs that have been developed and that inhibit blood vessel growth. Some cancer patients have experienced dramatic regression in their tumors using anti-angiogenic therapy.

We've saved the best for last. The great news is that God has created natural antiangiogenic foods that inhibit blood vessel growth to cancer clusters. These inhibitors are part of a healthy diet. Listed below are some of the more important natural inhibitors.

apples	dark chocolate	licorice
artichokes	garlic	maitake mushrooms
blackberries	ginger	nutmeg
blueberries	ginseng	olive oil
bok choy	grape-seed oil	oranges
broccoli	grapefruit	red grapes
brussels sprouts	green tea	parsley
cauliflower	lavender	pineapple
cherries	lemons	pumpkin
cranberries	kale	raspberries
soybeans	tomatoes	
strawberries	turmeric	

Usually, cancer is not discovered until it has metastasized and spread. This makes any treatment a little more difficult depending upon how much damage has been done. The above antiangiogenic foods do their best work in cancer prevention. However, there have been significant positive results for cancer and various other diseases by utilizing these cancer-fighting foods.

The Harvard School of Public Health did a prolonged study for twenty years following seventy-nine thousand men. They found that men who consumed two to three servings of cooked tomatoes per week reduced their risk of developing prostate cancer by 40–50 percent. [17]

The only exercise some people get is when they have the hiccups, sneeze, cut their nails, stand on their principles, get up and down from the table, jump to conclusions, and walk to the couch to watch their favorite TV program or play a video game.

Researchers have found that people who join a health club are fourteen times more aerobically active than those who do not belong to a club. They also have better cardiovascular health outcomes. [18] Health clubs provide professional help and advice, have quality exercise equipment, and create the opportunity to receive social support from others interested in health. An additional factor is the financial commitment, which encourages participation.

One of the major reasons for joining a health club is to lose weight. In one study it was found that male club members were able to lose about one and a half inches around their waists. There was a similar trend for women. [19]

The *New England Journal of Medicine* and the *Journal of the American Medical Association* both indicate that breast cancer risk was reduced by 30–40 percent for women exercising moderately. The risk dropped even further for women who exercised three to four hours a week. It is recommended that adults do thirty minutes of brisk walking five days a week. It is also suggested that they get seventy-five minutes of muscle-strengthening activities, like weight lifting. [20]

A vigorous five-mile walk will do more good for an unhappy but otherwise healthy adult than all the medicine and psychology in the world.
—Paul Dudley White

Within each cell structure are long strands of DNA called chromosomes. At the ends of chromosomes are *telomeres*, which function like bookends. Each time a cell divides, there's a tendency for the telomeres to become shorter.

Cells divide about fifty times before the telomeres become shorter. It's sort of like a pencil eraser that gets smaller each time it's used. Telomeres become a gauge by which we can measure the aging of a person.

In one study of women who *did not* get thirty minutes of exercise and were very sedentary with very little activity, it found that their telomeres were shorter than in women who exercised thirty minutes a day. It was estimated that this shortening added up to about eight years of aging within cells. The suggestion is that people who sit around a great deal show signs of aging more rapidly. That thought alone is enough to get you out of the comfort of your chair or bed. [21]

Another study indicated that changes in diet, exercise, stress management, and social support result in longer telomeres. The increased length of telomeres is associated with increased health, fewer illnesses, and longer life. [22]

Shorter telomeres are tied to many forms of cancer, stroke, vascular dementia, cardiovascular disease, obesity, osteoporosis, and diabetes. In one study of men with prostate cancer, they lengthened their telomeres with lifestyle changes. These included a plant-based diet (high in fruits and vegetables) and unrefined grains, a low-fat diet, moderate exercise (walking thirty minutes six times a week), stress reduction and schedule changes, breathing exercises, and meditation. The result was that they increased their telomere length by 10 percent over those did not make any of the above changes in lifestyle. [23]

What Exercise Does

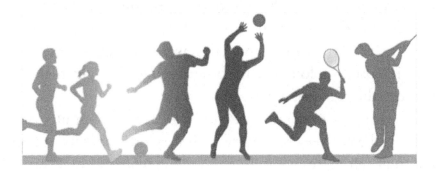

- Encourages the pituitary gland to release (feel-good painkiller) endorphins
- Reduces sensitivity to stress, anxiety, and depression
- Helps to prevent and treat dementia, Alzheimer's, and brain aging
- Increases activity in the temporal lobe and assists memory storage
- Reduces ADHD symptoms in children
- Assists in faster reaction time
- Reduces blood sugar levels and inflammation, which feed cancer growth

- Relieves fatigue resulting from disease or treatment
- Is useful for dealing with insomnia
- Strengthens the protection from relapse
- Aids in developing a positive mental attitude
- Creates an appreciation for nature when you exercise out of doors
- Fosters blood flow throughout the body and brain

In a fourteen-year study of men over sixty-five years of age who had prostate cancer and who exercised regularly, they had lower disease progression and a lower risk of dying from prostate cancer. [24] Researchers have shown that women who had breast cancer and began to eat a healthier diet and walk for thirty minutes six days a week reduced their risk of relapse by almost 50 percent. [25]

How about it?
Do you want to reduce the aging process?
Do these facts encourage you to exercise—
or do you want to just lie down until the thoughts pass?

Jim Hangstefer's Story

Jim was diagnosed with terminal brain cancer when he was twenty years old. Jim's doctors offered zero hope. They said they could maybe get a few more months of life with chemotherapy but he would still die of the cancer just a few months later.

Since doctors offered no hope, Jim and his wife put together a nutrition and vitamin program after reading a book for laypeople on vitamins and cancer. There was no guarantee or claim that the program would heal, treat, or prevent any disease.

Jim is now in his sixties and thriving. He has helped and encouraged thousands of people with cancer. Jim says that whole food products are the best way to deal with cancer. He took nutrients that contained carotenoids, cruciferous vegetables, and flavonoids. He also took a protein shake. He has had forty years of excellent, vibrant health with a nutrient program.

A ngela began to cry when she got the bad news.

"This is the final straw. I don't know how I can go on. I've got two kids in grade school. I just started a part-time job. My husband, Ralph, is in Afghanistan in the marines, and the oncologist just told me I've got stage three breast cancer. Who's going to take care of my children? How will we be able to afford the bills? And I'm afraid to die. I want to see my children get married. I want to enjoy grandchildren."

Life is filled with stress, difficulty, and pressure. We cannot escape its influence. We seem to be attacked in family relationships, with physical illness, in accidents, and through natural disasters. Cell phones, beepers, e-mail, faxes, Facebook, Twitter, long lines, road rage, noise, jam-packed schedules, meetings, overcrowding, barking dogs, and children with temper tantrums can confront us on a daily basis. Stressed passengers freak out when their flights are delayed or canceled.

A study published in the *British Journal of Science* found that women who experienced a severe stressful life event had a 1,500 percent increase in the risk of developing breast cancer. [26] Patrick Quillin, in his book *Beating Cancer with Nutrition*, states, "In my years of experience, about 90 percent of the cancer patients I deal with have encountered a major traumatic event one to two years prior to the onset of cancer. This is especially true of breast cancer patients. Not only can mental depression lead to immune suppression and then cancer, but there may be a metaphorical significance of the location of the cancer." [27]

A certain amount of stress is good and healthy for you. An upcoming test will cause you to study more diligently. Downhill skiing will sharpen your focus and coordination. This type of stress will add fun, excitement, and productivity to your life. However, living with too little stress, unproductive stress, or unhealthy stress can have a detrimental effect on you physically, emotionally, and spiritually. These types of stress create anxiety and depression.

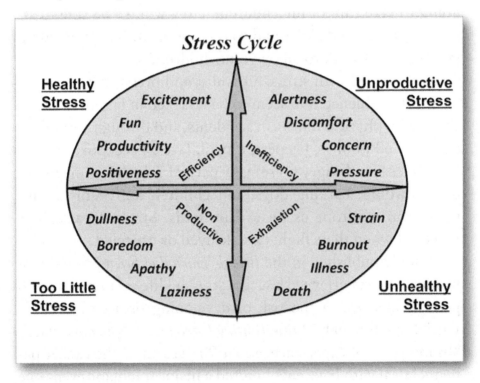

Emotional Signs of Stress

boredom
confusion
depression
detachment
disorientation
escape thoughts
feeling low
forgetfulness
sadness
sleep loss
uneasiness

impatience
insecurity
irritability
listlessness
nervousness
overexcitement
paranoia
quick-temperedness
worry

Visceral Signs of Stress

cold chills
cold hands
colitis
cramps
diarrhea
dry mouth
fainting
heart pounding

heartburn
light-headedness
moist hands
nausea
sweating
ulcers

Musculoskeletal Signs of Stress

arthritis

back pain

cramps

fidgeting

fist clenching

grinding teeth

headaches

jaw tightening

shaky hands

stiff neck

stuttering

tense muscles

tics

twitches

Other Signs of Stress

cold sores

compulsiveness

exhaustion

fatigue

frequent colds

hair twisting

hay fever

heart disease

high alcohol use

high caffeine use

high nicotine use

high sugar use

jumpiness

low sex drive

low spiritual life

nail biting

neglecting exercise

neglecting family

neglecting friends

neglecting fun

neglecting health

neglecting rest

no enthusiasm

no vigor

obesity

obsessiveness

Following is the famous Holmes and Rahe stress test. It will give you some idea of how much stress you may be encountering at this time in your life. Take a moment to review it and add up your score. Your total will indicate your susceptibility to illness. This is a result of your body's resistance being low because of the buildup of stress in your life for an extended period. Add points for each occurrence if there has been more than one during the last twelve months.

Life Event	Occurrences	Stress Value	Your Score
Death of a spouse		100	
Divorce		73	
Marital separation		65	
Detention in jail		63	
Death of close family member		63	
Major personal injury or illness		53	
Marriage difficulties		50	
Being fired from work		47	
Marital reconciliation		45	
Retirement from work		47	
Major change in health or behavior of family member		44	
Pregnancy		40	
Sexual difficulties		39	
Gaining a new family member by birth, adoption, moving in		39	

Major business readjustment, reorganization, bankruptcy	39	
Major change in financial status— better or worse	38	
Death of a close friend	37	
Changing to different line of work	36	
Major change in arguments with spouse—moreor less	35	
Taking out a major mortgage or loan	31	
Foreclosure on mortgage or loan	30	
Major change in responsibilities at work—promotion or demotion	29	
Children leaving home for marriage or school	29	
Trouble with in-laws	29	
Outstanding personal achievement	28	

Spouse begins or ceases work	26	
Beginning or ending school	26	
Major change in living conditions	25	
Revision of personal habits	24	
Troubles with boss	23	
Change in work hours or conditions	20	
Change in residence	20	
Changing to a new school	20	
Change in recreation—more or less	20	
Change in church activities	19	
Change in social activities	18	
Taking out a minor mortgage or loan	17	
Change in sleeping habits	16	
Change in family get-togethers	15	

Change in eating habits		15	
Vacation		13	
Christmas		12	
Minor violations of the law		11	

Your Total Stress Level Score

0–149: Healthy state of being, with normal stress

150–199: 37 percent chance of encountering illness in the near future

200–299: 50 percent chance of encountering illness in the near future

300 or more: 80 percent chance of encountering illness in the near future

So what does it all mean? If you have a score between 200 and 299, you need to make some minor adjustments to your lifestyle to insure a healthy immune system. If you have a score above 300, it's time for you to stop and take a look at your lifestyle. You need to consider making some major adjustments in the way you eat, sleep, and handle finances. Protect your health by eating more fruits and vegetables and less sugar and white flour. And you need to honestly evaluate your relationships at home, school, or work. Do you have broken relationships? Are you experiencing changes you have no control of? What is your present attitude at this time? Do you need some wise counsel from a friend, a relative, a minister, or some other trusted individual? Maybe it's an important time to consider the spiritual factors in your life. It's time to put on your big-boy or big-girl pants and deal with issues affecting your physical, mental, emotional, and spiritual health and well-being. It's something to think about.

Once we truly know that life is difficult—
once we truly understand and accept it—
then life is no longer difficult.
—M. Scott Peck

Dr. David Servan-Schreiber, in his book *Anticancer: A New Way of Life*, comments, "There is one cause of overproduction of inflammatory substances that is rarely mentioned when cancer is discussed: persistent feelings of helplessness, a despair that won't let up. This emotional state is accompanied by changes in the secretion of noradrenaline—known as the fight or flight hormone—and cortisol, the stress hormone. These hormones prepare the body for a potential wound, in part by stimulating the inflammation factors needed to repair tissues. At the same time, these hormones are also fertilizer for cancerous tumors, latent or already established." [28] Did you get it? Stress feeds and breeds cancer cells.

Dr. Servan-Schreiber is not alone in this area. Many studies have confirmed that ongoing stress can contribute to the development and progression of cancer. The famous Mark Twain addressed the stress of anger when he said, "Anger is an acid that can be more harm to the vessel in which it's stored than to anything on which it is poured." What's in your vessel today?

"It felt like all the air was sucked out of my body when my doctor told me, 'Tiffany, I have some difficult news. Our tests confirm that you have ovarian cancer.'

"I was in shock. I had so looked forward to having children, and that dream was suddenly destroyed. I felt all alone. My grief soon turned to anger. 'This is not right! It's not fair!' I wanted to scream, but deep down inside I knew it wouldn't help. The reality of what was happening to me began to settle in, and I didn't like it."

Each year thousands of men and women have to deal with the reality of some form of cancer attacking their bodies. This bad news is always a shock. It's followed by disbelief and accompanied by denial: "This can't be happening to me."

I can remember when our son-in-law got the news that he had skin cancer and had to have surgery to remove the growths. The reality of the situation affected not only him but our entire family. I could see the look of concern on his face when he got the doctor's diagnosis. He hesitated for a moment, took a deep breath, and said, "Why not me."

I was amazed at how quickly he moved to acceptance of the fact. Usually, it takes someone several weeks or months or even years to come to that position. I attribute his reaction to his strong spiritual faith.

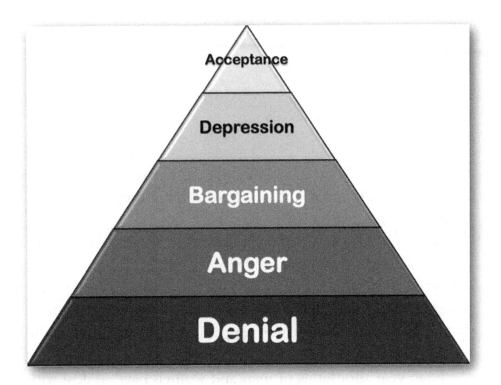

The normal grief cycle has five basic steps to it. First is the shock from the news you received, which is followed by *denial*. Denial can take the form of avoidance, confusion, fear, numbness, and even blame. The second step is *anger* over the situation. You may become frustrated, filled with anxiety, have displays of irritation, have feelings of embarrassment, and even feel shame. The third step involves some type of dialog and *bargaining*. This may involve you reaching out to others. You may have strong desires to share your story. The process begins a struggle for you to find meaning in what has just happened. When anger does not resolve the situation and bargaining doesn't help you, it often leads to *depression* and detachment. You may feel overwhelmed, experience the blahs, or lack energy to deal with the issue at hand. This creates a sense of helplessness, and you may feel like giving up. Eventually, you move toward acceptance. You begin to explore your options. You begin to make plans for the future. You make a determined effort to reinforce a positive attitude. Your focus turns from yourself and your problems and toward how you can help and encourage others.

You see, there's a difference between problems and facts of life. Problems are something you attempt to work on or change. Facts of life have to be accepted and made peace with. They are realities that are not going to change, and you have to accept them whether you like them or not.

For example, a couple of months before this writing, I cut off (amputated) my thumb in an accident. I was working with a radial-arm crosscut saw cutting some lumber. The piece of wood I was holding bucked and thrust my thumb in the route of the saw blade. In a split second, it was gone.

It took me a moment to fully process the reality of the situation. That moment ended quickly when I could see the blood and a missing thumb. I had to stop the bleeding, pick up the part of my thumb that was cut off, and drive two hours to the hospital.

My thumb is gone. No amount of denial or bargaining will bring it back. Anxiety, worry, anger, or depression will not make my thumb grow. My missing thumb is not a problem I can work on or change. It's simply a fact of life I have to accept and make peace with. The same is true of your cancer. It's a fact of life. Now it's up to you to accept it and make the best of what you can in the days ahead. Resistance to the fact of cancer will not help your attitude and or your ability accept to your affliction.

At the beginning of the early 1700s, Francois Fenelon addressed the subject of facing affliction. He said, "If we recognize the hand of God and make no opposition in our will, we have comfort in our affliction. Happy, indeed are these who can bear their sufferings in the enjoyment of this simple peace and perfect submission to the will of God! Nothing so shortens and soothes our pains as this spirit of nonresistance." The "spirit of nonresistance" is the same thing as learning to accept what we have no power to control.

I remember reading about Dr. Carl Menninger, who founded the Menninger Psychological Clinic in Topeka, Kansas. He was asked, "Dr. Menninger, how do you deal with depression?"

He said, "What you do is close all the windows in your home, shut all of your blinds, lock all of your doors…and then go across town and help someone who has worse problems than yours." It's a matter of attitude and focus. It's turning away from your own difficulties and looking to helping others. It's a great lifter of your spirit.

For many who hear they have cancer, it brings them face-to-face with the possibility of chemotherapy, surgery, radiation, and dying. It has been said that the true measure of life is reflected not in the number of years you live but in how you live those years. You may die on the sooner side, or you may live many more years. God is the only one who knows that answer. The question that remains is, how are going to live your life from this day forward? What will be your attitude?

Everything can be taken from a man but one thing:
the last of human freedoms—to choose one's attitude
in any given set of circumstances—to choose one's own way.
—Viktor Frankl

When it comes to health, it involves more than just the physical body. Man is made up of a body, a soul, and a spirit. Our bodies give us *physical contact* with the physical world. Our souls (which are made up of our minds, wills, and emotions) give us *self-consciousness* and *relational contact* with other people. And our spirits give us *God consciousness*.

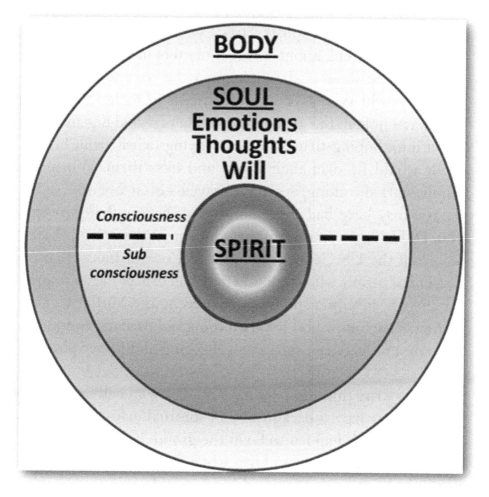

This book has, for the most part, been dealing with the body and how it functions with disease, especially cancer. But no matter how much time we spend addressing the mind, you still have emotions about cancer. It's impossible to separate the cancer from your emotions; they go hand in hand.

When it comes to the will, it's your choice mechanism. You will either choose to follow positive standards of buying, preparing, and eating healthy food, or you will choose to eat all the junk foods prepared for you sweet tooth.

What about your spirit? How's your spiritual life? Many choose not to think about spiritual matters until they're faced with death or some crisis. Remember the comment from the Second World War? "There's no atheists in foxholes." A foxhole was a hole in the ground that soldiers would dig and then crawl into, hoping that bullets and flying debris from bombshells would fly over their heads and miss them. When the bombs started coming, everyone prayed—even atheists.

You may have had the bombshell of cancer flying toward you. Did it cause you to think about spiritual matters? A survey from the US Centers for Disease Control found that 69 percent of people who were told they had cancer began to pray for their health. In a survey sponsored by the Moffet Cancer Center, they followed thirty-two thousand patients and found a strong link between spiritual well-being and better physical health.

As we write this book, we have no idea who will be reading it. Some may have a background in spiritual matters, and others may not. We happen to be in the group that has a spiritual background. We have found that when difficulties multiply and health issues increase, we need some outside help to deal with the issues that concern us.

That outside help comes from the Creator, who designed our wonderful and complex bodies. He knows how they work. He knows what foods are best for our health. And he knows we need assistance in dealing with our families, friends, neighbors, fellow workers, and strangers.

We appreciate you allowing us to share with you what we have found beneficial for us. We are fully aware that we both are sinners and our lives would be more difficult if it were not for our relationships with God. God helps when our emotions are a little out of control, when we think unwholesome thoughts, and when we say unloving things and do unloving acts toward others.

At a point in both of our lives, we came to a place where we realized we were running our lives and making a mess of them. We knew we needed outside help. That's when we came to a personal faith in Jesus Christ. We acknowledged Him as our Lord and Savior. We invited Him to come into our lives and change them. And change them He did. It's not been overnight. We have not become perfect. No one is perfect. But there have been many positive changes that have come about by our reading the Bible, praying, and going to church.

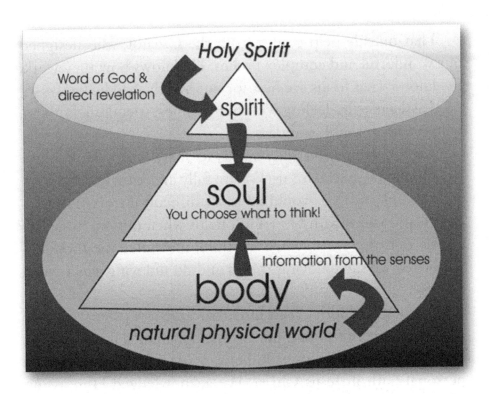

God sent His Holy Spirit to live in our bodies and light the candle of God consciousness that had been dark in our lives. He continues to enlighten and encourage us through the reading of the Bible. The Holy Spirit gives us wisdom about what to say and how to live a life that is kind, loving, and concerned for others.

We have no idea of your own personal spiritual background. We can only share with you the wonderful changes that have occurred since we invited Christ into our lives. If you have little or no resources in spiritual faith and hope, we would encourage you to consider Jesus. We became followers of Jesus.

We did that by a simple prayer of faith and said, "Dear Lord Jesus, I know that I'm a sinner, and I need Your help. I believe

You are the Son of God and You died for my sin on the cross. I believe You rose from the grave and You have conquered death. Please come into my life and change me. Thank You in advance for answering my prayer."

We realized that asking Jesus into our hearts would not keep us from all sickness. What it did do was give us help, instruction, and encouragement as we face difficult life issues. We would encourage you to do the same. Thank you for your openness and tolerance to allow us to share these important truths with you.

You can rest assured that we will be praying for you and others who will be reading this book, *Winning the Cancer Battle.*

The health care system in the United States is basically focused on symptoms of diseases or a cluster of symptoms.
Medical practice in reality becomes a chemical practice rather
than a total health practice. Drugs and surgery have become
the center of attention.

Unfortunately, our medical schools, hospitals, and govern-
ment health agencies and many doctors do not view nutrition
as playing a major role in the control of disease. For some
it doesn't play even a minor role. Often people who suggest
that nutrition is a key factor in battling disease are considered
"wacko" extremists that should be ignored until they go away.

There's no question there are highly educated and dedicated
men and women in the medical profession. The issue at hand
is one of broadening the perspective of health care. Medical
schools stress three major items: drugs, surgery, and radiation.
That's what they hammer into the minds of those who attend
training.

Years ago Abraham Maslow said, "If a person is familiar
with a certain, single subject, or has with them a certain, single
instrument, they may have a confirmed bias to believe that it is
the answer to or involved in everything. I suppose it is tempt-
ing, if the only tool you have is a hammer to treat everything as
if it were a nail."

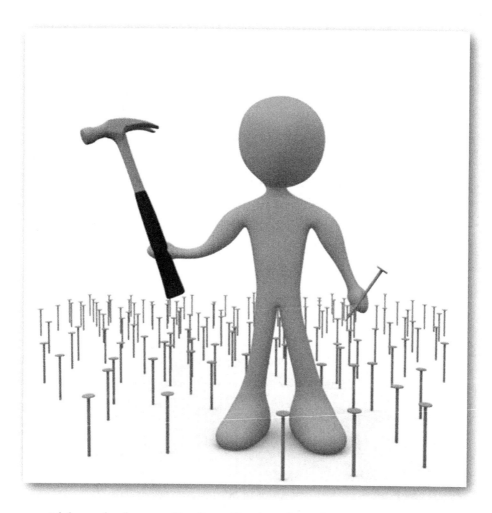

Although the medical profession has done good and wonderful things, you may be surprised to learn that medical malpractice and medical errors are the third-leading cause of death in the United States. A study conducted at Johns Hopkins revealed that 614,348 people a year died from heart disease, the number-one killer. Cancer is second, with over 551,000 deaths. Third in line were medical errors, which led to over 251,000 deaths. The medical errors included infections, poor hygiene, negligence, errors in diagnosis, giving the wrong medications to the wrong patient, and surgical errors, including removing the wrong organs or amputation of the wrong limbs. [29]

A great majority of medical practice is focused on individual symptoms or certain particular diseases. Often, because of time pressures or a lack of training, medical professionals fail to consider the larger picture of nutrition and lifestyle factors that contribute to the totality of ill health.

They become like the blind doctors examining the elephant. Each of the doctors focuses on one particular part of the elephant on which he or she has expertise.

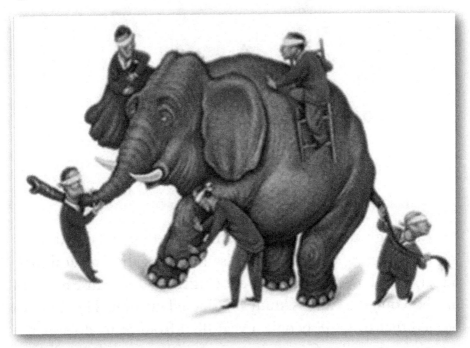

The ear doctor may have felt a warm ear and decided to examine further, only to discover a small tumor growing just inside the ear canal. Of course the inflammation needs to be reduced, and surgery is suggested to remove the tumor.

The nose doctor may have heard the elephant coughing and discovered it had been exposed to secondhand smoke and developed lung cancer. Since surgery in the lungs is difficult, the doctor prescribed chemotherapy.

The foot doctor found an old injury on the elephant and realized that it had become infected, which led to damaged cells. The damaged area had become susceptible to free radicals and developed a tumor that was beginning to spread. He was afraid the foot might need to be amputated, with radiation to follow.

The tail doctor could easily smell the symptoms of gastrological problems with the likelihood of colon cancer. Tests were administered, and a colonoscopy was recommended.

The skin doctor found a malignant melanoma and was concerned that it had already metastasized and spread to the lymph nodes in the neck area. Surgery, chemotherapy, and radiation were all recommended.

All the talented doctors were doing what they were trained for. They were dealing with symptoms. They didn't address the causes. For example, the lung doctor may suggest chemotherapy, but he says nothing about being exposed to secondhand smoke. The chemotherapy may help temporarily. But if the elephant doesn't stop his exposure to secondhand smoke, the lung cancer will return.

In 1662, doctors identified eighty-one different disease types. Today, the *International Statistical Classification of Diseases and Related Health Problems*, or ICD-10, lists over eight thousand diseases and conditions. Could it be that all these diseases have a similar cause and a similar cure: a significant change in the diet and lifestyle of the patient?

Before modern medicine, drugs were derived from plants and herbs in the human food chain. Today, the medical profession looks to drug chemicals as the answer to most human health issues other than old age, suicide, and accidents. The majority of modern drug chemicals are not found in the human food chain. They're created in scientific laboratories. Since they're not found in the human food chain, these drugs cause a host of side effects that the body attempts to deal with.

All you have to do is turn on your radio or television sets and listen to a multitude of commercials advertising various medications. Next time, listen carefully. They will quickly pass over a host of side effects of the medications, including lymphoma (cancer), depression, suicide, and death. Did you know that only the United States and New Zealand allow pharmaceutical companies to advertise directly to the public?

By the time symptoms of a disease have been diagnosed, the disease has already been in process for days, weeks, months, or even years. It's our opinion that it's better to deal with prevention rather than clean up a growing mess of ill health. That's why we have written this book. Which would you rather do: eat a whole food, plant-based diet or take drugs, have surgery, and receive radiation? It's your choice.

If we could give every individual the right amount of nourishment and exercise, not too little

and not too much, we would have found
the safest way to health.
—Hippocrates

Making positive lifestyle changes, like stopping smoking, reducing alcohol consumption, learning to handle stress, changing your diet to include less sugar and more fruits and vegetables, and getting proper exercise, will not only benefit you as a prevention of health issues; it will benefit you if you are in ill health right now.

I remember the story of the man who went to the doctor and told him, "Doc, every time I lift my arm it hurts!"

The doctor replied, "So don't lift your arm."

With regard to your health, is how you've been living helped you? Has your ill health been brought about by a poor diet and an unhealthy lifestyle? Then stop what you're doing. The bottom line in life is we do what we want to do. What do you want to do today?

You are not a victim of cancer and other diseases; you are a participant. The same is true for good health. You cannot sit around like a victim and expect to become healthy. You have to become a participant in your own health program. We would encourage you to make a determined decision to begin today. We believe you can do it.

He who has health has hope,
and he who has hope has everything.

The thought of cancer may be devastating, but remember that cancer is limited because of the following:

It cannot cripple *Love*.
It cannot shatter *Hope*.
It cannot corrode *Faith*.
It cannot destroy *Peace*.
It cannot kill *Friendship*.
It cannot suppress *Memories*.
It cannot silence *Courage*.
It cannot invade the *Soul*.
It cannot steal *Eternal Life*.
It cannot conquer the *Spirit*.

If I had cancer, this would be my action plan:

1. I would start by working with my doctor. I would make a list of questions I would like to ask him or her. I would not forget to check on the long and short-term effects of drugs, radiation, and surgery.

For the next six months, I would fanatically do the following:

2. I would educate myself on all possible alternatives. I would read books, watch documentaries, listen to cancer TED Talks, and search the Internet for answers. I would contact the person who gave me this book or one of the authors. I would get some psychological and spiritual counseling. I would be determined to keep a positive attitude.

3. I would become involved in a well-recommended detox program. I would attempt to remove as many free radicals and toxins from my body as possible.

4. I would start every morning with a tall glass of freshly squeezed lemon in warm water.

5. I would attempt to make my body more alkaline by changing my diet from acidic foods to alkaline foods. I would stop drinking soda drinks. I would be sure that I was taking calcium and minerals from a reputable company.

6. I would cut back on sugar foods like popcorn, cereal, red meats, ice cream, candy, pastries, white rice, potatoes, cooked carrots, white pasta, all sweeteners, honey, jam, ketchup, and so on.

7. I would begin to read labels of the foods I'm going to eat. I would attempt to eliminate foods made with toxic colorants, flavorings, and preservatives.

8. I would cook from scratch as much as possible. I would use only fresh washed and peeled organic food. I would eat more beans, lentils, and yams and plenty of vegetables. I would eat fresh fruit containing antioxidants, like all the berries, green apples, papaya, and grapefruit,

and reduce sweet fruits, like grapes and bananas. I would stop eating bacon and sandwich meats that contain nitrates and nitrites.

9. I would drink fresh vegetable juice comprising turmeric root, ginger, peeled lemon, peeled green apple, carrot, kale or swiss chard, cucumber, celery, and cabbage on a daily basis.

10. I would remove other toxins from my body, like shampoos, conditioners, body washes, shaving creams, toxic laundry detergents, toxic toothpastes, deodorants, some nail polishes, toxic lipsticks, and hand sanitizers.

11. I would attempt to fast daily from nine o'clock at night to eight in the morning and eliminate late-night snacks.

12. I would take megadoses of human-food-chain, organically grown, juice-extracted, GMO-free antioxidants and supplements that have a full spectrum of vitamin E, lipids and sterols, carotenoid families, bioflavonoid families, cruciferous families and garlic that has the full spectrum of allium and is target loaded.

13. I would get into a nonstress environment. I would avoid stress-producing movies and news. I would relax more and laugh more. I would schedule quiet times and mini vacations throughout the year.

14. I would begin an exercise program that would begin with a thirty-minute walk at least five times a week. I would increase the exercise program to forty-five minutes to an hour as I became more in shape.

15. I would drink plenty of alkaline water—but not with meals.

16. I would have a daily protein smoothie with either vegetables or various fruits.

17. I would eat plenty of salads with homemade salad dressing, like one cup of Bragg apple cider vinegar, one-third cup of olive oil, juice from one big lemon, salt, and pepper.

18. I would attempt to get more sunlight and enjoy God's magnificent creation.

19. I would begin breathing more deeply, thus helping to detox the lymph system.

20. I would spend more time with family and friends. I would attend church and began to focus on the spiritual side of life.

The Shopper's Guide to Pesticides in Produce from the Environmental Working Group (EWG.org) will help you determine which fruits and vegetables have the most pesticide residues and are the most important to buy organic. The Dirty Dozen plus One do not meet all the criteria but are commonly contaminated with pesticides toxic to the nervous system.

Dirty Dozen Plus One
1. Strawberries
2. Spinach
3. Nectarines
4. Apples
5. Peaches
6. Pears
7. Cherries
8. Grapes
9. Celery
10. Tomatoes
11. Sweet bell peppers
12. Potatoes
13. Hot peppers

Clean Fifteen
1. Sweet corn
2. Avocados
3. Pineapples
4. Cabbage
5. Onions
6. Sweet peas—frozen
7. Papayas
8. Asparagus
9. Mangos
10. Eggplant
11. Honeydew melon
12. Kiwi
13. Cantaloupe
14. Cauliflower
15. Grapefruit

Some sweet corn sold in the United States is produced from Roundup Ready genetically engineered seed stock. Most papaya is from genetically engineered seed stock.

On conventionally grown produce, insecticide can be applied externally or systemically. Systemic insecticides are put into the soil around the plant's root system and absorbed through the tissues and vascular system of the plant. When insects feed on the plant, they are killed by the insecticide. As a result, the vegetable/fruit is now contaminated with insecticide throughout that cannot be washed off.

Broccoli: Helps fight cancer: prostate, breast, vaginal, colon, and lung. To remove surfactants/pesticides, soak only (do not scrub).

Carrot: Great for eyes, cataracts, bad night vision, glaucoma. Contains calcium and beta carotene. Indigestible fiber: 2 percent absorption if eaten raw, 90 percent if juiced.

Cabbage: Benefits brain: helps cleanse stored toxins in fat cells (brain is made of fat cells). Helps stomach ulcers: drink within two minutes of juicing for enzymes to work on ulcers. Red cabbage has twice as many antioxidants as green. You get 10 percent of the enzymes when eating cabbage; juice it to get 90 percent of the enzymes.

Celery: Great for bones and nerves. Full of electrolytes, minerals, and salts.

Swiss chard: Full of nutrients (calcium, iron, zinc, minerals, and antioxidants) to help prevent osteoporosis, anemia, cardiovascular disease, and colon and prostate cancers; helps blood sugar control.

Beet: Great for boosting the immune system and red blood cell count; fights anemia; liver detox. Leaves are packed with nutrition, so juice them, but no more than a thumb-sized piece of the beet per person to avoid the high sugar content.

Cucumber: Detoxifies eyes, mouth; freshens breath; helps with water retention in the extremities, the heart, and so on. Must use original stocky cucumber, not English or Japanese varieties. Clean by rubbing with vegetable cleaner; then juice with the skin on.

Apple: Tangier fruit has more vitamin C and antioxidants; sweeter fruit has more calories; seeds have antioxidants and bioflavonoids. Peel store-bought apples to remove wax coating, even organic. If homegrown and pesticide-free, leave the skin on to increase vitamin content.

Ginger: Source of electrolytes; great for clear brain, indigestion, heartburn, stomach ulcers, upset tummy, and diarrhea; an immunity booster and a cancer fighter; increases alkalinity.

Turmeric: Fights cancer, boosts immunity, helps digestion, mental health, diabetes, and kidneys; increases alkalinity; appetite suppressant.

Pineapple: Helps reduce uric acid and sore joints and protects kidneys. In some countries, it is called pyne (pain) apple. Scrub the whole pineapple, top included, with a brush and diluted vegetable wash, rinse, and then remove top. Juice the whole fruit—skin, core, and all.

Orange: For all oranges, whether purchased or homegrown, remove the zest (orange skin) with a potato peeler; keep the white pith, as nutrients dissipate into the pith within weeks of harvesting.

Tropical Juice: one orange, one apple, and a one-inch slice of pineapple. For pain and kidney protection.

Lemonade: three medium-size apples and a quarter of a lemon, peeled. This is a tasty sugar-free lemonade, a great thirst quencher and cleanser.

Tropical Fruit: one apple, one orange, and a slice of pineapple. Orange assists in kidney health, and pineapple facilitates in dealing with uric acid, sore joints, and kidney disorder.

Great Veggie Juice: one apple, three carrots, three inches of celery, a sliver of cabbage, two inches of cucumber, about six buds and stems of broccoli, one-quarter slice of a large beet along with two beet leaves, and kale.

Blood Buster: two oranges, peeled, and a quarter of a beet. This is packed with nutrients, especially if you have a low red blood count.

Fruit Punch: one kiwi, one apple, one cup of grapes, one cup of berries, one slice of pineapple, one pear, and one orange, peeled. This makes a great juice.

Orange Special: one orange, peeled, one apple, and a two-inch slice of pineapple (use more if not sweet enough). If you would like to turn this juice into a meal-replacement smoothie, add two scoops of vanilla protein powder.

Basic Smoothie: one cup of water, one cup of ice, two scoops of chocolate or vanilla protein powder. Blend until mixed.

Strawberry Smoothie: two strawberries, one banana, half a pear, one spoon of plain yogurt, quarter cup of milk, quarter cup of water, and two scoops of vanilla protein powder. Blend until smooth.

Strawberry Delight Smoothie: —One half cup of ice, half cup of water, three strawberries, one banana, six grapes, two scoops of vanilla protein powder. (If you freeze the grapes and strawberries, it will make the drink colder. If you freeze the banana, you will not need to use ice.) Blend until smooth.

Kiwi Smoothie: one kiwi, one banana, half a pear, one spoon of plain yogurt, quarter cup of milk, quarter cup of crushed ice, and two scoops of vanilla protein powder. Blend until smooth.

Cinnamon-Banana Smoothie: cinnamon to taste, one banana, half cup of water, half cup of ice, and two scoops of chocolate protein powder. Blend until mixed.

Orange Smoothie: one orange, peeled, one peach, half cup of water, half cup of ice, and two scoops of vanilla protein powder. Blend until mixed.

Almond-Mint Smoothie: fresh mint, almonds, half cup of water, half cup of ice, and two scoops of chocolate protein powder. Blend until mixed.

Berry Smoothie: half cup of mixed berries, one banana, half cup of water, half cup of ice, and two scoops of chocolate protein powder. Blend until mixed.

Vegetable Smoothie: half cup of lettuce tops, one tablespoon of sesame seeds, one cup of water, one cup of ice, and two scoops of vanilla protein powder. Blend until mixed.

Resources to Educate Yourself

YouTube

- "My Potato Project" (2 Minutes)
- *Seeds of Death* (movie)
- "TED Talks: Jamie Oliver"
- "The World According to Monsanto"
- "5 GMO Myths Busted"
- *Fat, Sick & Nearly Dead* (movie)
- *The Beautiful Truth* (movie)
- "How to be an Effective Juicer"
- "Sugar: The Bitter Truth" (Dr. Lustig)
- "Fat Chance: Fructose 2.0"
- "The Marketing Madness:"
- "Are We All Insane?"
- "The Quest for the Cures"

Documentaries (Netflix, etc.)

- *The Future of Food*
- *Hungry for Change*
- *The Human Experiment*
- *Food Inc.*
- *Food Matters*
- *Farmageddon*
- *GMO OMG*

Apps

- Fooducate
- noGMO
- ShopNo/GMO

- GMO Tester
- Dirty Dozen (EWG)
- Skin Deep
- EWG Food Scores

Websites

- EGWG.org
- NonGMOProject.org
- NonGMOShopping
  Guide.com
- WHFoods.org
- GreenMedInfo.com
- HealthierEating.org
- ImageAwareness.com
- WhatonMyFood.org
- GoodEarthMill.com
- http://off-grid.info/
  food-independence/
  heirloom-seed-suppli-
  ers.html
- EatWild.com
- FoodRenegade.com

Books/Reports

- *Prescription for
  Nutritional Healing*—
  Phyllis A. Balch

- *Your Body's Sign
  Language*—James W.
  McAfee
- *Fresh Vegetables & Fruit
  Juices*
- *Colon Hygiene: The Key
  to a Vibrant Life*—N. W.
  Walker
- *Wheat Belly*—William
  Davis
- *Whole: Rethinking the
  Science of Nutrition*—T.
  Colin Campbell
- *Anticancer: A New
  Way of Life*—David
  Servan-Schreiber
- *The China Study*—T.
  Colin Campbell
- *The Definitive Guide
  to Cancer*—Lise N.
  Alschuler and Karolyn
  A. Gazella
- *Beating Cancer with
  Nutrition*—Patrick
  Quillin

The Roots of Cancer

(1)   David Servan-Schreiber—*Anticancer: A New Way of Life*—page 4

(2)   Patrick Quillin—*Beating Cancer with Nutrition*—page 65

The Amazing Immune System

(1)   David Servan-Schreiber—*Anticancer: A New Way of Life*— page 143

The Big *C* Word

(1)   https://search.aol.com/aol/search?s_it=webmail-searchbox&q=whatismetastasis-newsmedicallifesciences

(2)   Patrick Quillin—*Beating Cancer with Nutrition*—page 57

(3)   https://search.aol.com/aol/search?s_it=sb-top&v_t=webmail-searchbox&q=obesity- centerfordiseasecontrol

Avenues of Prevention

(1)   https://search.aol.com/aol/search?s_it=webmailsearchbox&q=newsmedical. netwhat%20is%20metastyasis

(2) Lise N. Alschuler and Karolyn A. Gazella—*The Definitive Guide to Cancer*—page 18

(3) Patrick Quillin—Beating Cancer with Nutrition—page 92

(4) Lise N. Alschuler and Karolyn A. Gazella—*The Definitive Guide to Cancer*—page 68

(5) T. Colin Campbell and Thomas M. Campbell—*The China Study*—page 139

(6) Lise N. Alschuler and Karolyn A. Gazella—*The Definitive Guide to Cancer*—page 27

(7) David Servan-Schreiber—*Anticancer: A New Way of Life*—page 111

(8) https://search.aol.com/aol/search?s_it=sb-top&v_t=webmail-searchbox&q=garlicand+cancerpreventionnational+cancer+institute

(9) https://search.aol.com/aol/search?s_it=sb-top&v_t=webmail-searchbox&q=somevitaminsupplementsraiseriskofcancerinmenresearchtheguardian

(10) https://search.aol.com/aol/search?s_it=sb-top&v_t=webmail- searchbox&q=newstudyinjournalofamericanmedicalassociationsays organicconsumersassociation

(11) https://search.aol.com/aol/search?s_it=sb-top&v_
t=webmail- searchbox&q=alphalipoicacid%3Athemultita
skingsupplementnaturalnews.com

(12) Patrick Quillin—Beating Cancer with Nutrition—page 276

(13) Patrick Quillin—Beating Cancer with Nutrition—page 285

(14) https://search.aol.com/aol/search?s_it=sb-top&v_t=webmail-se
archbox&q=synergistictoxicityoffoodadditivesinratsfedadietlow
indietaryfiberjournaloffoodscience

(15) https://search.aol.com/aol/search?s howmuchwaterdoyou
havetodrinkto"undo"cola-carlagoldenwellness

(16) https://search.aol.com/aol/search?s_it=sb-home&v_
t=webmail-&q=robertg.allen-yourhealthisindanger

(17) https://search.aol.com/aol/search?s_it=sb-top&v_
t=webmail-&q=tomatoesandprostatecancer-harvard-
healthpublications

(18) https://search.aol.com/aol/search?s_it=sb-top&v_
t=webmail-&q=toimprovehealthandexercisemore%2Cge
tagymmembership-sciencedaily

(19) https://search.aol.com/aol/search?s_it=sb-top&v_
t=webmail-&q=toimprovehealthandexercisemore%2Cge
tagymmembership-sciencedaily

(20) Lise N. Alschuler and Karolyn A. Gazella—*The Definitive Guide to Cancer*—page 52

(21) https://search.aol.com/aol/search?s_it=sb-top&v_t=webmail-&q=telomersandaging-understandingcellular-aging

(22) https://search.aol.com/aol/search?s_it=sb-top&v_t=webmail-&q=telomersandaging-understandingcellular-aging

(23) https://search.aol.com/aol/search?s_it=sb-top&v_t=webmail-&q=telomersandaging-understandingcellularaging

(24) Lise N. Alschuler and Karolyn A. Gazella—*The Definitive Guide to Cancer*—page 75

(25) Lise N. Alschuler and Karolyn A. Gazella—*The Definitive Guide to Cancer*—page 272

(26) Patrick Quillin—Beating Cancer with Nutrition—page 48

(27) Patrick Quillin—Beating Cancer with Nutrition—page334

(28) David Servan-Schreiber—*Anticancer: A New Way of Life*—page47

(29) https://search.aol.com/aol/search?s_it=sb-top&v_t=webmail-&q=john%27shopkinsstudysuggestsmedicalerrorsarethirdleadingcauseofdeathinunitedstates

About the authors

L ouis Smith is a certified nutrition consultant, certified holistic nutrition consultant, and certified John Maxwell coach. His own cancer went into remission twenty-seven years ago. Now, Smith travels the world and speaks to audiences of up to eleven thousand people about the link between nutrition and health. He is also the author of *Plan to Succeed*.

Bob Phillips, PhD, is a certified nutrition and wellness consultant and licensed marriage and family therapist. He cofounded the Pointman Leadership Institute, which presents seminars about leadership and ethics in over seventy countries. Phillips is also director emeritus for Hume Lake Christian Camps. He has written over 130 books on a variety of subjects, including his Babylon Rising series, *How to Deal with Annoying People*, *Overcoming Anxiety & Depression*, *7 Seconds to Success*, and *Optimal Health and Wellness*. If you have difficulty finding beneficial and healthy supplements, you can e-mail me at bob2hume@gmail.com and I will be happy to assist you.

Made in the USA
Middletown, DE
07 June 2020